Practice Long Cases for the Part B Final FRCR Examination

JENNIFER DAVIDSON
MRCS FRCR
Specialist Registrar in Radiology
University Hospital Southampton

BETH SHEPHERD
MRCS FRCR
Specialist Registrar in Radiology
University Hospital Southampton

and

SUNDERARAJAN JAYARAMAN
MRCP FRCR
Consultant Radiologist
St Richard's Hospital, Chichester

Radcliffe Publishing
London • New York

Radcliffe Publishing Ltd
33–41 Dallington Street
London
EC1V 0BB
United Kingdom

www.radcliffehealth.com

British Library Cataloguing in Publication Data

A catalogue record for this book is available from the British Library.

ISBN-13: 978 184619 550 1

The paper used for the text pages of this book is FSC® certified. FSC (The Forest Stewardship Council®) is an international network to promote responsible management of the world's forests.

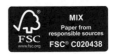

Typeset by Darkriver Design, Auckland, New Zealand
Printed and bound by Hobbs the Printers, Totton, Hants, UK

Contents

About the DVD

AMI-VIEW is a software package distributed as a companion to the book *Practice Long Cases for the Part B Final FRCR Examination* by Jennifer Davidson, Beth Shepherd and Sunderarajan Jayaraman, published by Radcliffe Publishing Ltd. The principal software author is Jim O'Doherty.

Windows users

Minimum requirements (for good operation): Windows XP, 2GHz Processor, 2GB RAM, >500 MB hard disc space.

1. Insert the DVD.
2. Find the file labelled "MCRInstaller.exe".
3. Double click this file and follow the onscreen instructions to install to the default directory: C:\Program Files\MATLAB\MATLAB Compiler Runtime\v715\bin\win32.

   If you choose to install to a different directory, please see the extra information below.
4. It should take approximately 170 MB of disc space. This file installs the environment for the program to operate.

You only need to perform steps 1–4 *one time only*.

5. Double click the file "runme.bat" which launches the main program.
6. The program requires the DVD to be kept in the drive at all times.
7. The next time you want to run the program, simply double click the "runme.bat" file. *You will need the DVD in the drive every time you use the program.*

Program is compatible with Windows 7, XP, Vista. No other Windows versions were tested.

Extra Windows information

Please use this information only if you have changed the default installation directory from that specified in Step 3.

   If you choose not to install to the default directory (C:\Program Files\

MATLAB\MATLAB Compiler Runtime\v715\bin\win32) then you need to change the folder specified in the "runme.bat" file to the folder that you installed to.

Mac users

Minimum requirements: Mac OS X 10.6.4 (Snow Leopard) and above with Apple Java for Mac OS X Update 2 and above.

1. Insert the DVD.
2. Find the folder "MCR_R2012a_maci64_installer".
3. Double click on the file "InstallForMacOS".
4. Accept the terms and licences and follow the on-screen instructions for installing.
5. Please install the program to the default location which should be: "Applications/MATLAB/MATLAB_Component_Runtime/v717".

    If you choose to install to a different directory, please see the extra information below.

You need to perform steps 1–4 *one time only.*

6. To run the program, simply double click the file labelled "run_AMI_ View.command".
7. The program should then run automatically. *You will need the DVD in the drive every time you use the program.*

Extra Mac information (advanced users)

Please use this information only if you have changed the default installation directory from that specified in Step 5.

Open a terminal window (you can find it in Utilities/Terminal) and navigate to the directory on the DVD. You will need to type something like cd ../../Volumes/PracticeCases.

This navigates you from your user profile to "Users" to "Volumes" and onto the DVD. Verify this by typing "ls" (without quotations) and you should see the contents of the DVD.

Then type the following:

./run_AMI_View.sh <INSTALLDIR>

where <INSTALLDIR> is the *full* pathname to the installed directory

To use the program

Simply click (once) on a Paper and the corresponding cases will appear on the selection box to the right.

Clicking on the case will display thumbnails of the series available for study.

Clicking on a thumbnail once will cause it to be displayed in a viewer.

Tools such as zooming and automatic windowing and slice scrolls are included in the viewer where necessary.

Please contact jim.odoherty@gmail.com for technical information.

Legal disclaimers

In using the DVD-ROM and all the included software, you acknowledge and accept this Disclaimer of Warranty:

We encourage readers to communicate with us concerning significant modifications to the software, so that they may be incorporated in future versions of the software, with proper credit to the contributors.

About the authors

Jenny Davidson started her radiology training on the Manchester scheme before transferring to the Wessex rotation, where she is currently a Specialist Registrar. Her areas of interest include nuclear medicine and musculoskeletal and oncology imaging. Outside of work, free time is mostly taken up with foreign travel and watching live cricket or music.

Beth Shepherd also trained in radiology on the Wessex scheme and is currently a Specialist Registrar. Her areas of interest include oncology and abdominal imaging. She has organised the medical student teaching for the past few years and she also enjoys travel and watching rugby (often together).

Sunderarajan Jayaraman is a Consultant Radiologist at St Richard's Hospital, Chichester, where he has worked for the past 8 years.

Acknowledgements

Thank you to Jim O'Doherty, Medical Physics, Division of Imaging Sciences, King's College London, and Lisa O'Brien, Superintendent Radiographer, Nuclear Medicine, St Richard's Hospital, Chichester, for their help and support in developing the software and providing the data.

Thanks in addition to Dr Howard Portess, Dr Catherine Grierson and others from University Hospital Southampton who proofread the text.

To our families

List of abbreviations

A&E	Accident and Emergency department
ACL	anterior cruciate ligament
AIDS	acquired immune deficiency syndrome
AVN	avascular necrosis
AVM	arteriovenous malformation
CT	computed tomography
DIP	desquamative interstitial pneumonia
DMSA	dimercaptosuccinic acid
FIGO	International Federation of Gynaecology and Obstetrics (classification system)
FLAIR	fluid-attenuated inversion recovery
FNH	focal nodular hyperplasia
FRCR	Fellowship of the Royal College of Radiologists
GBM	glioblastoma multiforme
HIV	human immunodeficiency virus
HSV	herpes simplex virus
IAM	internal auditory meatus
Ig	immunoglobulin
MAG3	mercaptoacetyltriglycine
MDT	multidisciplinary team
MIBG	metaiodobenzylguanidine labelled to iodine-123
MM	multiple myeloma
MRA	magnetic resonance angiography
MRI	magnetic resonance imaging
PA	psoriatic arthritis
PAP	pulmonary alveolar proteinosis
PCL	posterior cruciate ligament
PD	proton density
PE	pulmonary embolism
PET-CT	positron emission tomography and computed tomography
RA	rheumatoid arthritis
RCC	renal cell carcinoma

RCR	Royal College of Radiologists
RN	reflux nephropathy
SPECT	single photon emission computed tomography
STIR	short T1 inversion recovery
TCC	transitional cell carcinoma
TNM	Tumour, nodes, metastases (cancer staging system)
UIP	usual interstitial pneumonitis
US	ultrasound
UTI	urinary tract infection
VIBE	volume interpolated breath-hold examination
V/Q	ventilation–perfusion
VUR	vesicoureteral reflux
WHO	World Health Organization

Introduction

The FRCR (Fellowship of the Royal College of Radiologists) Part 2B is a challenging examination consisting of:
- an oral examination
- a rapid reporting session
- a reporting session (also known as the 'long cases').

More details about the examination, its structure and its rules can be found on the Royal College of Radiologists (RCR) website (www.rcr.ac.uk). This examination is the culmination of years of hard work and training, and the RCR rightly makes it a difficult and robust examination to challenge trainees and ensure they have reached an appropriate standard. Preparation is absolutely vital for success and we hope this book provides a useful opportunity to hone essential skills.

To create this book we have drawn upon our recent experiences of revising for and sitting the 2B examination. This can be a very stressful time and the multiple parts of the examination rely on different and distinct techniques. Preparation for the oral examination and the rapid reporting session is extremely well catered for, and there are plentiful opportunities to practice examination techniques. In our experience the reporting session was much more difficult to prepare for, because of a lack of relevant textbooks and because of very limited opportunities to sit good practice papers. This 'gap' inspired us to write this practice paper book. We hope this book will give you the opportunity to practise this component of the exam, by printing off the sample blank answer paper and using the digital images, all of which are available on the accompanying DVD, to recreate examination conditions.

The examination

The reporting session in the examination lasts for 60 minutes, during which time the candidate will be asked to write a report on each of six cases. Each case may include up to four digital images or imaging sequences – these may include plain films, CT, ultrasound, radionuclide and MRI scans. A brief case history and other relevant clinical data will be provided. The cases vary in complexity and difficulty but all cases carry equal weighting in the marking scheme; some require more time for analysis and reporting than others. Reports should be brief, relevant and legible. It is recommended that candidates use bullet points rather than long sentences. Under no circumstances should a question be left blank – there will always be something that a candidate can write.

Each candidate will be provided with a formatted answer book in which to write reports on *all* six cases. The format, as outlined on the RCR website, is as follows.

Observations

In this section, you should record your observations on the films from all the imaging studies available to you, including relevant positive and negative findings.

Interpretation

Here you should state your interpretation of the observed findings; for example, describe whether the mass or process you observe is benign, malignant or infective rather than neoplastic, and give your reasons.

Often 'Observations' and 'Interpretation' are answered as one section, as demonstrated in one of the sample answers outlined later in this introduction, as this avoids repeating information. However, if it suits the candidate, they can be answered separately.

Principal diagnosis

Based on your interpretation you should attempt to come to a single diagnosis. If this is not possible, then state here which diagnosis you feel is most likely and then list other possibilities, in order of likelihood, in the differential diagnoses section.

Differential diagnoses

For some cases there will be no differential diagnoses, in which case it is preferred to leave this section blank rather than include inappropriate differentials. In others cases, you may feel that you wish to include a few; these should be limited in number and brief. In your report you should indicate why you feel these were less likely than your main or principal diagnosis.

Management

In this section you should indicate any further appropriate investigations or clinical management. For example, if you diagnose a patient with a subdural collection, then urgent referral is needed if there is evidence of brain compression. Similarly, if you make a diagnosis of an abscess or tumour, indicate if a drainage or biopsy is appropriate.

Sample answers

CASE 1
A 10-month-old child seen unconscious in the A&E department

Observations and interpretation
- A non-contrast head CT shows an extra-axial fluid collection on the left side of the brain. The shape of this suggests that it lies within the subdural rather than the subarachnoid space. It contains both high and low attenuation material, indicating that it is likely to represent an acute or chronic subdural haematoma. Midline shift is seen with compression of the left lateral ventricle. No skull fracture is seen on these images.
- A chest radiograph shows fractures of the left sixth and seventh ribs posterolaterally, with evidence of callus formation indicating healing. There are also fractures of the right eighth and tenth ribs posteriorly, but no associated callus or periosteal new bone, suggesting that these fractures have occurred very recently. These findings suggest that these rib fractures have occurred at different times. The lung fields are clear.

Main diagnosis
Non-accidental injury

Differential diagnoses
Consider accidental trauma (this appears unlikely in view of the posterior rib fractures of different ages)

Further management
- The patient needs an urgent neurosurgical opinion and the child protection service must be alerted.
- A skeletal survey should be performed to look for other fractures and to ensure that there is no evidence of any other skeletal abnormality such as osteogenesis imperfecta.

CASE 2
A 2-year-old child with a painful left hip

Observations
Observations on abdominal radiograph:
- ill-defined lytic lesion of the left femoral neck with associated periosteal new bone formation;
- calcification in the right upper quadrant;
- possible paravertebral mass around the L1 vertebral body.

Observations on skeletal scintigram (bone scan):
- areas of increased uptake in the left sixth, seventh and eighth and the right fourth, fifth and eighth ribs, the right humerus and the left femur;
- possible areas of increased activity in the region of calcification seen on the abdominal radiograph.

Interpretation
- The lesion in the left femoral neck has the appearance of an aggressive lesion suggestive of malignancy. Infection appears unlikely.
- The calcification in the right upper quadrant could relate to the liver, gallbladder, kidney or adrenal gland. In the context of possible malignancy, this is likely to relate to a malignancy in the adrenal gland.
- The possible paravertebral soft tissue mass will need further investigation with cross-sectional imaging but it may indicate intraspinal extension of an adrenal tumour.
- The areas of increased activity on the bone scan suggest widespread skeletal metastases.

Main diagnosis
Neuroblastoma in right adrenal region with bone involvement and possible intraspinal extension

Differential diagnoses
- Adrenal carcinoma can occur rarely in this age group; it may calcify but it is unlikely to extend intraspinally.
- Wilms' tumour is intrarenal, it only occasionally calcifies and it rarely metastasises to bone, so it should not give these appearances.

Further management
- An ultrasound scan would confirm whether the calcified mass lies within the adrenal gland.
- An MRI scan, MIBG scan and skeletal scintigram would be required for staging and monitoring response to treatment.
- Bone marrow aspiration and catecholamine estimation are usually also performed.
- A biopsy may also be required.

These sample answers are adapted from the RCR website (www.rcr.ac.uk/content.aspx?PageID=713).

Timing

Time management is absolutely essential and sufficient time should be allocated to report each case adequately. Always time yourself in the examination, and practice doing this at home. In total you have 10 minutes for every question, but it is advisable that you should aim to spend 7–8 minutes on each question; this allows you to allocate extra time to longer or more challenging questions, gives you time to read over the questions and answers, and ensures that you will not run out of time. When the examiner says stop writing, they mean stop writing.

Marking scheme

Another challenging part of examination preparation is interpretation of the marking scheme. We found this particularly frustrating when preparing for the examination ourselves. There are guidelines provided by the college, but these can be open to interpretation depending on the individual cases and it can be very difficult to 'score' yourself accurately. We hope that this book will allow you to be more confident that your answers are meeting the required standards.

The college marking scheme

Mark	Outcome
4	Bad fail
5	Fail
6	Pass
7	Good pass
8	Excellent

In general, if the principle diagnosis is identified correctly then the candidate will have passed that question (a mark of 6 or above). The quality of the observations and interpretations, differential diagnoses and management then dictate whether the candidate scores 6, 7 or 8.

If the quality of the candidate's observations and interpretations are good and the principle diagnosis is mentioned in the differential diagnoses, then the pass mark will almost certainly be awarded. Even if the principle diagnosis has not been mentioned at all but the quality of the other sections is excellent, then the candidate may still be awarded a pass.

Conversely, candidates will be penalised for incorrect statements, lack of discrimination in conclusions and for suggestions of clinically inappropriate additional investigations and management. This will obviously become important in answers that are deemed a borderline pass.

Candidates are not required to pass every question, but if one question is failed then a score above the pass mark (i.e. 7 or 8) will have to be achieved on another question to compensate.

Using this book

The digitalisation of the examination has been a great success and is much more applicable to clinical practice than before. This digitalisation also tests new skills such as image manipulation and processing of larger quantities of information in an examination setting. On the accompanying DVD are the digital images for 12 practice papers, as well as specially produced software to enable viewing of the images on a personal computer. Regarding the MRI studies, only selected sequences that give the relevant information have been included, rather than the entirety of a particular study, so as to fit within the time limitations of the examination. Single printed images are included in the printed section of the book to allow quick reference or for those with limited access to a computer, although we strongly suggest that the practice papers be used in conjunction with the DVD. On these single printed images, while we have tried to include representative images, obviously it may not be possible to make all the necessary observations. Also on the DVD is a sample blank answer paper that can be printed off and used for the practice papers.

For each question there is a model answer provided – this answer would score an 8 in the examination. It is against this model answer that users should mark their own practice papers, using the guidance outlined earlier in this introduction.

Of note, there may be variations in interpretation that have not been included in the model answer, as we have tried to make the book as succinct and usable as possible. Additionally, there may be management suggestions that have not been explicitly mentioned but which may well be valid. Therefore, we urge users to exercise common sense when applying marking schemes.

The discussion session section for each case is designed to give a brief overview of the imaging findings and of the main pathologies discussed. It is beyond the scope of this book to give detailed reviews; these can be sought by using the references and the standard textbooks.

In addition to the named references that follow the discussion, we have utilised the standard textbooks the most candidates have access to. These are:

- *Radiology Review Manual*, by WF Dähnert (7th edition; Lippincott, Williams & Wilkins; 2011)
- *Primer of Diagnostic Imaging*, by Ralph Weissleder, Jack Wittenberg, Mukesh G Harisinghani and John W Chen (5th edition; Elsevier; 2011)
- *Aids to Radiological Differential Diagnosis*, by Stephen Chapman and Richard Nakielny (5th edition; Saunders Elsevier; 2009).

The named references are the ones we found useful in our background reading. These were chosen either as review articles, which include useful imaging overviews, or to illustrate best clinical practice.

Top tips

- **Time each individual question.** Remember you have 10 minutes maximum per question, try to aim for 7–8 minutes per question.
- **Never ever leave a question unanswered.** There is always something you can write. Even if you cannot spot an abnormality use the clinical details as a guide. You can always give pertinent negatives, formulated some differential diagnoses and give a sensible management plan.

- **If you are struggling, move on and then come back later.**
- **Be logical.** This will not only help the examiner marking your paper but will also help you formulate an good answer.
- **Be succinct.** Use bullet points and be legible.
- **Be safe.** In the management section communicate that you are a safe radiologist. For example, if you think it is an emergency, say it is an emergency.
- **Don't panic.** Remember that you do not need to pass each question. Be confident in your preparation.

We hope you find using this book a valuable addition in your examination preparation. We wish you luck for the big day and all the best for your future careers.

Jenny and Beth
November 2012

Paper 1

Case A
History
A 6-year-old boy who fell and now has pain in his left forearm

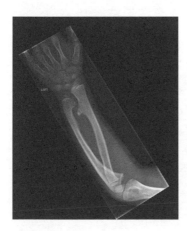

Figure i Radiograph of the left forearm

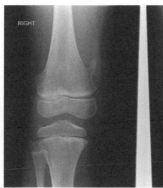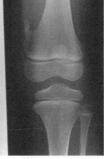

Figure ii Radiograph of the knees

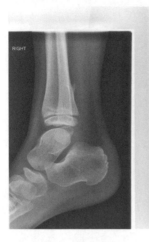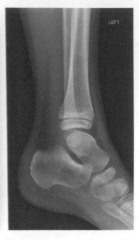

Figure iii Radiograph of the ankles

Observations and interpretation
Radiograph of the left forearm:
- exostoses (osteochondromas) are seen arising from the left distal radius and ulna;
- these extend away from the joint;
- bowing of the radius and ulna;
- the ulna is shortened with angulation of the lateral aspect of the physis, causing a pseudo-Madelung deformity;
- no fractures or irregularity of the exostoses are appreciated.

Radiograph of the knees and ankles:
- further multiple exostoses extending away from the joint;
- no evidence of fracture or irregularity of the exostoses.

Main diagnosis
Multiple exostoses consistent with diaphyseal achalasia or hereditary multiple exostoses

Differential diagnoses
None – this is an Aunt Minnie appearance

Further management
- If clinical suspicion of fracture persists, then MRI could be useful to look for radiographically occult injury.

- MRI can also be useful to look at size and position of the cartilage cap and any potential impingement of adjacent structure.
- Discuss and consider the familial connotations.

Discussion

Diaphyseal achalasia is an autosomal dominant condition characterised by multiple metaphyseal exostoses (also known as osteochondromas) that point away from the joint. This condition is seen slightly more commonly in males and it is usually discovered by the age of 12 years. Diagnosis is usually via plain film and can often be an incidental finding, particularly if there is no family history of the condition. Unfortunately, 40% of those with diaphyseal achalasia have short stature, due to the formation of exostoses at the expense of longitudinal bone growth; up to one-half of those with the condition will have abnormal shortening of an extremity.

Exostoses are most commonly seen around the knee and are usually in the appendicular skeleton. In the upper limb, they are associated with pseudo-Madelung deformity, dislocation of the radial head, shortening of the fourth and fifth metacarpals and supernumerary digits. In the lower limb, abnormalities include coxa valga, genu valgus and Erlenmeyer flask deformity of the distal femur.

Complications other than those related to bone growth include an increased risk of fracture of the exostoses, which can be secondary to only minimal trauma. Impingement of local structures by the exostoses can also cause symptoms. There is also a risk of transformation of the cartilage cap of the exostoses into a malignant chondrosarcoma, although this would be highly unusual in the paediatric population. A 2 cm upper limit for cartilage cap thickness is used to distinguish between benign osteochondromas and secondary chondrosarcomas; this gives sensitivity and specificity nearing 100% in both CT and MRI. Both modalities are also used to identify occult injury and local impingement if clinically indicated.

Reference

Bernard SA, Murphey MD, Flemming DJ, *et al.* Improved differentiation of benign osteochondromas from secondary chondrosarcomas with standardized measurement of cartilage cap at CT and MR imaging. *Radiology*. 2010; **255**(3): 857–65.

Case B

History

A 64-year-old male with ongoing intermittent abdominal pain and a previous history of right hemicolectomy

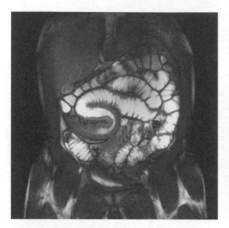

Figure i Coronal HASTE MRI   **Figure ii** Coronal truFISP MRI

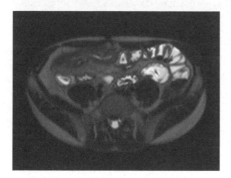

Figure iii Axial HASTE MRI

Observations and interpretation

MRI enterography of the small bowel (coronal HASTE, coronal truFISP and axial HASTE sequences):

- the terminal ileum just proximal to the ileocolic anastomoses is abnormal;
- the affected segment shows wall thickening, loss of normal features and some narrowing of the lumen;
- this area does not show significant enhancement, suggesting chronic inflammation;

- local lymphadenopathy;
- no skip lesions;
- the jejunum looks satisfactory, as does the rest of the imaged bowel and solid organs;
- no discrete collections, gallstones, sacroiliitis, evidence of fistula formation or other complication.

Main diagnosis
Chronic Crohn's disease affecting the distal ileum

Differential diagnoses
- Other causes of terminal ileum inflammation that include infection (*Yersinia*, tuberculosis) and malignant causes of bowel wall thickening (lymphoma) should be considered.
- Ulcerative colitis should not be considered, as there is no evidence of colitis in the remnant colon.

Further management
- Gastroenterology referral and discussion at the MDT meeting.
- Consider ultrasound of the abdomen as a baseline of bowel wall thickening, as this is a useful modality in assessing response to treatment.
- Consider endoscopy for full luminal assessment and biopsy for histological diagnosis.

Discussion
Crohn's disease is an inflammatory bowel disease of uncertain aetiology. It is characterised by granulomatous inflammation with asymmetric and discontinuous involvement of the entire gastrointestinal tract. In addition to the gastrointestinal manifestations, there is a myriad of extra-enteric disease.

In Crohn's disease, bowel involvement is frequently segmental – the diseased segments are referred to as 'skip lesions'. The earliest changes affect the mucosa, producing aphthoid ulceration and lymphoid hyperplasia, which progresses to longitudinal and horizontal mucosal ulceration, and then to transmural ulcer formation, resulting in sinuses, fistulas and perienteric abscesses. In the more chronic phase, inflammation leads to fatty infiltration of the bowel wall and fibrofatty proliferation in adjacent mesenteric fat. Wall fibrosis causes strictures and consequent bowel obstruction. Acute and chronic changes may coexist within the same diseased segment.

Depending on the clinical scenario, there are multiple modalities that are used to investigate Crohn's disease. These routinely include ultrasound, CT, fluoroscopy studies and MRI. CT plays an invaluable role in the evaluation of acutely ill patients with Crohn's disease, particularly when there is concern for high-grade obstruction, perforation or abscess.

MRI enterography is increasingly utilised for investigation and problem solving in the management of Crohn's disease. MRI enterography offers the advantages of multiplanar capability and lack of ionising radiation, and it can assess both luminal and extraluminal disease. It is particularly useful in patients with a high suspicion of small bowel disease. MRI enterography allows evaluation of bowel wall contrast enhancement, wall thickening and oedema – findings useful for the assessment of Crohn's disease activity. MRI enterography can also depict other pathological findings such as lymphadenopathy, fistula and sinus formation, abscesses and abnormal fold patterns. Even subtle disease manifestations may be detected if adequate distention of the small bowel is achieved, although endoscopic and double-contrast barium small bowel techniques remain superior in the depiction of changes in early Crohn's disease (e.g. aphthoid ulceration). The choice of enterography over enteroclysis is a practical one. Enteroclysis has been shown to more accurately depict early disease and the number of involved segments, whereas enterography is more time efficient for radiologists and other staff, since nasojejunal tube placement is not required.

Typical changes of Crohn's disease include ileal involvement, fat wrapping, wall thickening, linear and aphthoid ulcers, fistulisation, skip lesions and 'cobblestoning'. However, several MRI enterographic findings are associated with increased disease activity, including wall thickening greater than 4 mm, intramural and mesenteric oedema, mucosal hyperaemia, wall enhancement (and enhancement pattern), transmural ulceration and fistula formation, vascular engorgement and inflammatory mesenteric lymph nodes (often with hyperenhancement). There is an emerging majority opinion that MRI imaging enhancement patterns reliably help to discriminate between active and inactive disease.

References

Hafeez R, Punwani S, Boulos P, *et al*. Diagnostic and therapeutic impact of MR enterography in Crohn's disease. *Clin Radiol*. 2011; **66**(12): 1148–58.

Tolan DJ, Greenhalgh R, Zealley IA, *et al*. MR enterographic manifestations of small bowel Crohn disease. *Radiographics*. 2010; **30**(2): 367–84.

Case C

History

A 40-year-old female with non-specific lower abdominal pain

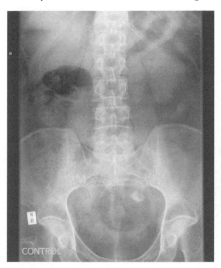

Figure i Abdominal radiograph

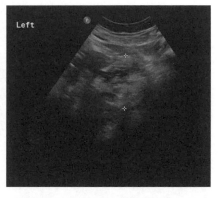

Figure ii Transabdominal ultrasound (left pelvis transverse section)

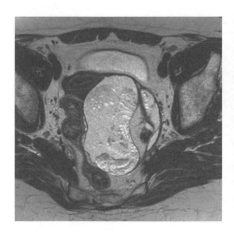

Figure iii MRI T2 axial

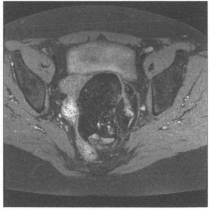

Figure iv MRI STIR axial

Observations and interpretation

Abdominal radiograph:
- normal bowel gas pattern;
- in the left hemi-pelvis is a rounded low-density structure containing a focus of calcification.

Transabdominal ultrasound:
- 6 cm containing heterogeneous echogenicity lesion in the left adenexa, potentially containing fat;
- no definite calcification identified.

MRI of the pelvis (T1, T2 and STIR axial):
- left adnexal mass;
- well-defined low-signal rim and internal heterogeneous high signal on T1 and T2 which suppresses out, consistent with fat;
- focal area of low signal in the left lateral wall is 'tooth shaped' and is in keeping with calcification;
- uterus, right ovary, bladder and rectum unremarkable;
- no lymphadenopathy or free fluid.

Main diagnosis

Mature cystic teratoma or dermoid – uncomplicated

Differential diagnoses
- These appearances are characteristic of a dermoid.
- Other rare differentials would include ovarian lipomas or lipoleiomyomas.

Further management

This would not usually require biopsy, as the imaging appearances are characteristic.

There are no features to suggest complication such as haemorrhage or torsion; therefore, this may not be the cause of the lower abdominal pain – consider other investigations to ensure alternate pathology has not been missed.

Discussion

Mature cystic teratomas (a more appropriate term than the commonly used 'dermoid cysts') are cystic tumours composed of well-differentiated derivations from at least two of the three germ cell layers (ectoderm, mesoderm and endoderm). They affect a younger age group (mean patient age, 30 years) than epithelial ovarian neoplasms and are the most common ovarian mass in children. They are bilateral in about 10% of cases. Most mature cystic teratomas are asymptomatic. Abdominal pain or other non-specific symptoms occur in the minority of patients. They can tort, bleed or compress other structures to cause symptoms.

The gross pathologic appearance of mature cystic teratomas is character-istic. Hair follicles, skin glands, muscle and other tissues lie within the wall. There is usually a raised protuberance projecting into the cyst cavity known as the Rokitansky nodule. Ectodermal tissue (skin derivatives and neural tissue) is invariably present. Mesodermal tissue (fat, bone, cartilage, muscle) is present in over 90% of cases, and endodermal tissue (e.g. gastrointestinal and bronchial epithelium, thyroid tissue) is seen in the majority of cases. Adipose tissue is present in up to three-quarters of cases and teeth in up to a third of cases.

Mature cystic teratomas are usually recognised at ultrasound, although ultrasound diagnosis is complicated by the fact that these tumours may have a variety of appearances. A hyperechoic area is a highly predictive feature of a dermoid, particularly when it is associated with distal acoustic shadowing. Hyperechoic lines and dots, sometimes called the dermoid mesh, are also very predictive. Less common but also characteristic are a fluid-fluid level with the more echogenic fluid located in a non-dependent position and floating globules. The demonstration of any two or more of the aforementioned features in a mass is particularly predictive of a dermoid. Calcification, often due to bone or a tooth, occurs in some dermoids, but cannot be used alone as definitive evidence of a dermoid, since other neo-plasms can also calcify. Other manifestations include a cystic lesion with a densely echogenic tubercle (Rokitansky nodule) projecting into the cyst lumen, a diffusely or partially echogenic mass with the echogenic area usu-ally demonstrating sound attenuation owing to sebaceous material and hair within the cyst cavity and multiple thin, echogenic bands caused by hair in the cyst cavity. Rarely, a dermoid will not have any of these characteristic ultrasound features.

The diagnosis of mature cystic teratoma at CT and MRI imaging is fairly straightforward because these modalities are more sensitive for fat. At CT, fat attenuation within a cyst, with or without calcification in the wall, is diagnostic for mature cystic teratoma. A floating mass of hair can sometimes be identified at the fat-fluid interface.

At MRI imaging, the high signal of fat on T1 and T2 must be distin-guished from intracystic haemorrhage. The imaging appearance on T1- and

T2-weighted images is therefore mimicked by some haemorrhagic lesions – most prominently, endometriomas. Chemical shift, gradient echo and fat suppression sequences can help distinguish between mature cystic teratoma and endometriomas.

Mature cystic teratoma can be associated with complications from rupture, malignant degeneration (only 1% or 2% and usually in those over 60 years of age), or most commonly torsion. It is mainly larger lesions that are at risk of torsion. Torsion, even in chronic cases, does not eradicate the fatty elements. Findings suggestive of torsion include deviation of the uterus to the twisted side, local inflammatory change, engorged blood vessels on the twisted side, a mass with a high-signal-intensity rim on T1-weighted MRI images, a low-signal-intensity torsion knot, blood vessels that drape around the mass and complete absence of enhancement.

Reference

Outwater EK, Siegelman ES, Hunt JL. Ovarian teratomas: tumor types and imaging characteristics. *Radiographics*. 2001; **21**(2): 475–90.

Case D

History
A 2-year-old with wrist deformity

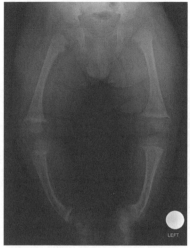

Figure i Radiograph of the lower limbs

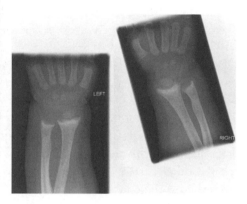

Figure ii Radiograph of the wrists

Observations and interpretation
Radiograph of the lower limbs:
- metaphyseal flaring and cupping;
- the tibiae are bowed;
- the metaphyses at the hips are also flared.

Radiograph of the wrists:
- soft tissue swelling;
- metaphyseal cupping, flaring and splaying.

Main diagnosis
Rickets

Differential diagnoses
There are a number of less common differentials for both leg bowing and metaphyseal flaring. Leg bowing can also have developmental causes, including congenital bowing and osteogenesis imperfecta. Other causes of metaphyseal flaring include lead poisoning and storage diseases.

Further management
Discussion with the Paediatricians for review of diet and family history

Discussion
There are a number of causes of bowing in infants and children, developmental, congenital and acquired. Developmental, or 'physiological' bowing is associated with varus angulation centred at the knee, thickening of the medial tibial cortices and tilted ankles. Blount's disease or tibia vara is associated with genu varum and depression of the proximal tibia medially. Congenital bowing can occur and is seen as cortical thickening along the concavity of the curved tibia.

The underlying pathophysiology of rickets is that of deficient mineralisation of normal osteoid and disruption of the normal development and mineralisation of growth plates. The most common forms are vitamin-D deficient (hypophosphatasia) and nutritional rickets. There is bone softening that leads to bowing on weight bearing. The changes are seen on plain radiographs at the sites of rapid growth and involve the metaphyses, with cupping, fraying and splaying occurring with growth and continued weight bearing. Sites of rapid growth include the proximal humerus, distal radius, distal femur and both ends of the tibia. Treatment is dietary and medical unless the bowing is severe, when surgical management, such as valgus osteotomies, may be considered.

Metaphyseal flaring and cupping is also seen with achondroplasia, as well as short, thick long bones. Anterolateral bowing is typically seen with neurofibromatosis, often with focal narrowing and sclerosis or cystic change at the apex of the curve. Bone softening, seen with osteogenesis imperfecta, also leads to bowing of long bones.

Reference
Cheema JI, Grissom LE, Harcke HT. Radiographic characteristics of lower-extremity bowing in children. *Radiographics*. 2003; **23**(4): 871–80.

Case E

History

60-year old male patient presents with right-sided weakness

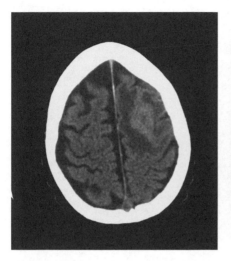

Figure i Pre-contrast CT of the brain

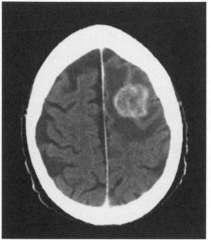

Figure ii Post-contrast CT of the brain

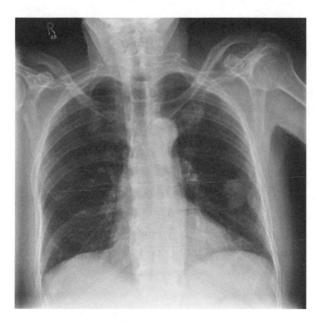

Figure iii Chest radiograph

Observations and interpretation
Pre- and post-contrast CT of the brain:
- there is a hyperdense rounded lesion in the left frontal lobe, with surrounding white matter vasogenic oedema;
- post-contrast, this area shows avid peripheral enhancement with central low density;
- there is mild local sulcal effacement but no midline shift;
- the basal cisterns are patent;
- the venous sinuses enhance normally;
- no further parenchymal lesions;
- no destructive bone lesions.

Chest radiograph:
- lobulated soft tissue mass at the left lower zone, which is suspicious for a bronchial neoplasm;
- the lesion is solitary;
- normal cardiomediastinal contour and bones.

Main diagnosis
Brain metastasis secondary to bronchial carcinoma, in view of the lesion on the chest radiograph and the extensive white matter oedema

Differential diagnoses
Primary bronchial carcinoma with haemorrhagic infarction

Further management
- Referral to Chest physicians and Lung MDT meeting
- Further staging CT to assess for mediastinal lymph nodes and thoracic or abdominal metastatic disease

Discussion
Hyperdense lesions on CT are generally caused by neoplasia composed of high cellular density, including cerebral lymphoma, pineoblastoma, neuroblastoma, medulloblastoma. Metastases from primary malignancies, such as melanoma, bronchogenic, colon and breast carcinoma, may also be hyperdense. MRI of these lesions is typically of low signal intensity on T2-weighted images, due to high nucleus-to-cytoplasm ratio and hence less free water. Contrast enhancement indicates breakdown of the blood–brain barrier, which is seen in other pathological states, in addition to malignancy,

including inflammation, subacute infracts, post-operative gliosis and radiation necrosis.

There are a number of causes of intracranial haemorrhage. Haemorrhagic venous or arterial infarction, hypertensive haemorrhage, underlying vascular or arteriovenous vascular malformation, coagulopathies or underlying neoplasm may cause intracranial parenchymal haemorrhage.

Intracranial tumours are a recognised cause of intracranial haemorrhage, with underlying pathogenesis including tumour necrosis, vascular invasion and neovascularity. Glioblastomas, in the primary malignancy group, are the most common tumour associated with haemorrhage. Haemorrhagic metastases occur in the context of bronchogenic, thyroid, melanoma, choriocarcinoma and renal cell carcinoma. It may be difficult to distinguish between primary haemorrhage and underlying malignancy on CT, in the context of a solitary lesion. MRI findings of intratumoural bleeds include a more complex, heterogeneous pattern, delayed evolution of blood products (possibly from intratumoural hypoxia), enhancing components (although primary haematomas may develop ring enhancement in the subacute phase), increased and persisting peri-lesional oedema relative to primary haemorrhage, absent or incomplete haemosiderin ring at 2–3 weeks. A follow up MRI scan between 3 and 6 weeks after the initial study may help to clarify the diagnosis and obviate the need for a surgical biopsy.

In the context of multiple haemorrhagic parenchymal lesions, haemorrhagic metastases should be a key consideration. A possible differential would be multiple cryptic arteriovenous malformations, which can occur either *de novo* or secondary to radiotherapy, and which have a similar imaging appearance, apart from the extent of surrounding vasogenic oedema.

References

Olsen WL. Central nervous system neoplasms and tumor like masses. In: Brant WE, Helms CA. *Fundamentals of Diagnostic Radiology*. 3rd ed. Philadephia, USA: Lippincott Williams & Wilkins; 2007. pp. 122–55.

Rowley HA. Cerebrovascular disease. In: Brant WE, Helms CA. *Fundamentals of Diagnostic Radiology*. 3rd ed. Philadephia, USA: Lippincott Williams & Wilkins; 2007. pp. 86–121.

Case F

History

A 70-year-old female, previous cerebrovascular accident

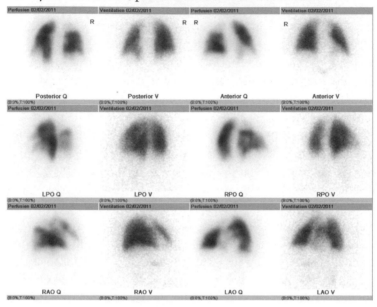

Figure i Ventilation–perfusion scan

Observations and interpretation

Ventilation–perfusion (V/Q) scan:

- multiple segmental and subsegmental perfusion defects, affecting the left posterior base, right upper lobe and the right middle lobe, indicating a high probability of acute pulmonary embolus;
- the ventilation study demonstrates uniform uptake bilaterally.

Main diagnosis
Bilateral pulmonary embolus

Differential diagnoses
None

Further management
- Review of previous imaging to assess whether this is an acute or chronic embolus
- Urgent report to the referring clinicians

Discussion
When describing V/Q scans, it is important to consider the following:
- if there are defects on the ventilation or perfusion images;
- if they are matched or mismatched;
- if there are perfusion defects, whether they are segmental, subsegmental or non-segmental.

The typical description of pulmonary embolism (PE) on V/Q scans is of segmental or subsegmental, mismatched perfusion defects. It is important to remember to consider the chest radiograph when interpreting the V/Q scan, as pre-existing pathology, such as chronic airways disease, asthma, consolidation or pleural effusions can affect the diagnostic yield of the study.

The original data for analysis of V/Q imaging was based on the Prospective Investigation of Pulmonary Embolism Diagnosis study. This study was performed in 1985 but gathered extensive clinical data, which produced the following conclusions.
- High probability V/Q scans were reliable indicators for PE.
- Normal or near normal scans were reliable to exclude disease.
- A high clinical probability with high probability scan equated to 96% accuracy in diagnosing PE (and the same degree of accuracy for low clinical and scan probabilities).

Subsequently, revised criteria were produced, which confirmed the following points.
- A single moderate size mismatch segmental defect was unlikely to be low probability.
- Multiple matched defects could be described as low probability if there were no other perfusion defects present.

25

- Two or segmental perfusion defects was satisfactory for high probability.

The Prospective Investigative Study of Acute Pulmonary Embolism Diagnosis studied 890 patients with suspected PE. This study found that clinical assessment combined with perfusion scan evaluation confirmed or excluded PE in the majority of patients, without the need for ventilation imaging. Most hospitals tend to have a protocol whereby patients with a normal chest radiograph undergo a perfusion scan only and an intermediate outcome generates a CT pulmonary angiogram, and patients with an abnormal chest radiograph undergo a CT pulmonary angiogram. This arrangement provides the best diagnostic yield.

Reference

Miniati M, Pistolesi M, Marini C, *et al.* Value of perfusion lung scan in the diagnosis of pulmonary embolism: results of the Prospective Investigative Study of Acute Pulmonary Embolism Diagnosis (PISA-PED). *Am J Respir Crit Care Med.* 1996; **154**(5): 1387–93.

Paper 2

Case A

History

A preterm neonate on the paediatric intensive care unit with multiorgan dysfunction

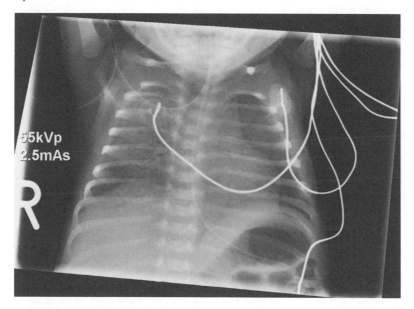

55kVp
2.5mAs

R

Figure i Chest radiograph

Observations and interpretation

Chest radiograph:
- bilateral ground-glass shadowing;
- small volume lungs;
- satisfactory position of lines and tubes;

- normal cardiomediastinal contour;
- no pneumothorax or pneumomediastinum.

Main diagnosis
Respiratory distress syndrome or surfactant deficiency disease

Differential diagnoses
- Pulmonary infection: neonatal infections are most commonly group B *Streptococcus*, but this is more likely to be asymmetrical.
- Meconium aspiration: this can be seen in preterm infants but is most common in those who are post term. Classically, coarse linear and irregular opacities are seen and the lungs become hyperexpanded.
- Transient tachypnea of the newborn is seen in term infants but can have similar radiological findings to surfactant deficiency disease.

Further management
- Inform the referring team
- Consider surfactant therapy if not already initiated

Discussion
Surfactant deficiency disease is seen in premature infants because of lung immaturity and lack of adequate surfactant production. Symptoms usually arise soon after birth but the maximum radiological findings are seen at 12–24 hours. Classically, there is a fine granular pattern in the lungs and air bronchograms, later on the heart borders, and diaphragmatic outlines can become obscured. Small lung volumes are seen because of micro-atelectasis.

Most infants make a full recovery after surfactant therapy. Some infants unfortunately encounter complications of the disease process or treatment. Affected infants often require ventilation therapy and complications of this positive pressure ventilation can be seen radiographically; these include interstitial emphysema, pneumomediastinum and pneumothorax. Complications can also ensue after oxygenation with bidirectional or right to left shunting through the ductus arteriosus, which may lead to pulmonary oedema and cardiomegaly.

Reference
Agrons GA, Courtney SE, Stocker JT, *et al*. From the archives of the AFIP: lung disease in premature neonates; radiologic-pathologic correlation. *Radiographics*. 2005; **25**(4): 1047–73.

Case B

History

A 65-year-old female with acute-onset distended abdomen and vomiting

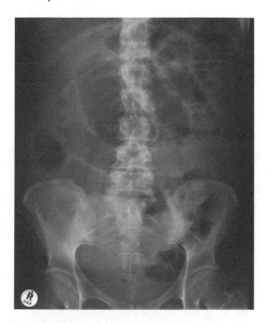

Figure i Abdominal radiograph

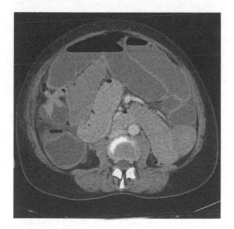

Figure ii Portal venous phase CT

Observations and interpretation

Abdominal radiograph:
- dilated loops of bowel, mainly small;
- no evidence of pneumoperitoneum.

CT of the abdomen and pelvis (portal venous phase):
- apple core stenotic lesion in the proximal transverse colon highly suspicious for malignancy just beyond the hepatic flexure; proximal to this is large and small bowel obstruction;
- the colon distal to the obstruction is collapsed;
- no pneumoperitoneum but there is a small amount of free fluid;
- no lymphadenopathy;
- the liver contains several simple cysts but no evidence of metastases;
- the rest of the solid organs are unremarkable; an intrauterine contraceptive device is noted in the uterine cavity;
- the lung bases are clear bar atelectasis;
- no suspicious bony lesions.

Main diagnosis

Stenosing colonic carcinoma in the proximal transverse colon causing proximal large and small bowel obstruction

Differential diagnoses

There is no real differential diagnosis. The stenotic lesion is carcinoma until proven otherwise.

Further management

- Inform the referring team
- Urgent referral to the appropriate oncological MDT meeting
- CT of the chest should be performed for full staging
- May be useful to obtain tumour markers, particularly carcinoembryonic antigen

Discussion

Colorectal cancer is a common malignancy that results in significant morbidity and mortality. The majority of cases occur on the left colon, usually rectosigmoid. Right-sided cancers can present late, as they often have non-specific symptoms.

CT is essential in the diagnosis and assessment of patients with colorectal cancer because it can demonstrate regional extension of tumour as well as adenopathy and distant metastases. On CT, colorectal cancer typically appears as a discrete soft tissue mass that narrows the colonic lumen. Colorectal cancer can also manifest as focal colonic wall thickening with or without luminal narrowing. Additionally complications associated with the primary tumour such as obstruction, perforation and fistula formation can be visualised with CT. At CT, local extension of tumour appears as an extracolic mass or simply as thickening and infiltration of pericolic fat. Extracolic spread is also suggested by loss of fat planes between the colon and adjacent organs.

Metastases are usually haematogenous or lymphatic, the liver being the most common site. Hepatic metastases are best visualised during the portal venous phase of liver enhancement; features include reduced enhancement compared to the background liver, low attenuation and poor definition. They can occasionally be cystic, or undergo cystic transformation after chemotherapy, which can make assessment more challenging. Smaller lesions are harder to characterise and can often be occult. In more equivocal lesions or if hepatic surgery/ablation treatment is being considered then contrast enhanced MRI routinely is used for characterisation and location of lesions. Hepatic metastectomies are becoming increasingly common, as up to 15% of cases have surgically resectable disease and there is a proven survival advantage. Percutaneous ablation therapies can also be utilised to treat sites of metastatic disease. Other common sites of metastases from colon cancer include the lungs, adrenal glands and bones.

TNM STAGING OF COLORECTAL CANCER

Primary tumour (T)

TX = primary tumour cannot be assessed

T0 = no evidence of primary tumour

Tis = carcinoma in situ

T1 = tumour invades the submucosa

T2 = tumour invades the muscularis propria

T3 = tumour invades through the muscularis propria into the subserosa
or into non-peritonealised pericolic or perirectal tissues

T4 = tumour directly invades other organs or structures or perforates the
visceral peritoneum

Regional lymph nodes (N)

NX = regional lymph nodes cannot be assessed

N0 = no regional lymph node metastasis

N1 = metastasis in 1–3 pericolic or perirectal lymph nodes

N2 = metastasis in ≥4 pericolic or perirectal lymph nodes

Distant metastasis (M)

MX = distant metastasis cannot be assessed

M0 = no distant metastasis

M1 = distant metastasis

CT is heavily utilised for initial staging but is also critical for identifying recurrences and assessing response to treatment.

Reference

Horton KM, Abrams RA, Fishman EK. Spiral CT of colon cancer: imaging features and role in management. *Radiographics*. 2000; **20**(2): 419–30.

Case C

History

A 36-year-old female being investigated for subfertility

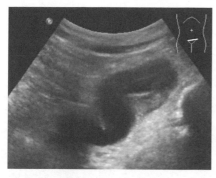

Figure i Transvaginal ultrasound (left iliac fossa)

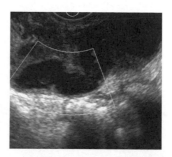

Figure ii Transvaginal ultrasound (left iliac fossa)

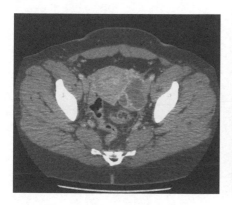

Figure iii Portal venous phase CT

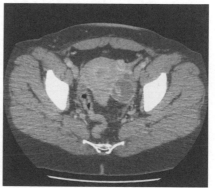

Figure iv Portal venous phase CT

Observations and interpretation

Transvaginal ultrasound:

- anteverted normal uterus;
- within the left adnexa is a tubular, thick-walled structure, some low-level internal echoes are noted within the structure;
- no free fluid seen.

CT of the abdomen and pelvis (portal venous phase):

- corresponding to the ultrasound appearances, an abnormal thick-walled fluid-filled tubular structure is demonstrated in the left iliac fossa;
- the ovaries are not clearly identified on either side;
- unremarkable uterus;
- no free fluid or lymphadenopathy;
- no further significant findings within the abdomen/pelvis;
- lung bases are clear;
- no suspicious bony lesions.

Main diagnosis
Left hydrosalpinx

Differential diagnoses
- Pyosalpinx/haematosalpinx
- Abnormal loop of small bowel

Further management
- Referral to a Gynaecologist and Gynaecology MDT meeting
- Ensure screen for pelvic inflammatory disease and pregnancy test has been performed
- Consider MRI to rule out lesion not appreciated on CT

Discussion
The term hydrosalpinx is used to describe a dilated fallopian tube filled with fluid. Blockage usually occurs at the fimbriated end of the fallopian tube and is commonly caused by adhesions from infectious or inflammatory processes. The most common causes are pelvic inflammatory disease and endometriosis; among women with these conditions, approximately 8% develop hydrosalpinx. Other causes include iatrogenic lesions – for example, post-surgical adhesions, tumours of the pelvis and rare intra-abdominal infections such as tuberculosis.

At ultrasound, a hydrosalpinx appears as a thin-walled, tubular, serpiginous structure, which is usually identified separately from the ovaries, although it may be attached by adhesions. Other ultrasound findings include small polypoid lesions of the wall that can appear similar to the spokes of a cogwheel on transverse images and a 'waist sign' or concentric indentation of the cystic structure has been reported to be quite specific for hydrosalpinx. In patients with chronic hydrosalpinx, submucosal folds are flat and nodular, an appearance known as the 'beads on a string' sign. When ultrasound findings are equivocal, MRI or CT imaging is usually performed. At CT, care should be taken with patients who have not ingested oral contrast material, because the small bowel may mask or mimic dilated fallopian tubes.

The imaging features of pyosalpinx are similar to those of hydrosalpinx; however, pyosalpinx is more likely to be bilateral. Other features of pyosalpinx include fallopian tube wall thickening, thickened uterosacral ligaments, oedema of the presacral fat and associated small bowel ileus. The ultrasound features of pyosalpinx are similar to those of simple hydrosalpinx; therefore, it is important to be familiar with the patient's clinical history and to recognise the clinical features of sepsis that are indicative of pyosalpinx.

Haematosalpinx results from obstruction and dilatation of the fallopian tubes by blood products. It most commonly occurs in the context of endometriosis, although a tubal ectopic pregnancy, pelvic inflammatory disease, adnexal torsion, malignancy, and trauma can also cause tubal bleeding. Altered blood products within a haematosalpinx demonstrate homogeneous low-level echoes at ultrasound, high attenuation at CT, and high signal intensity at T1-weighted fat-suppressed MRI imaging. These blood products may cause adhesions to fold or pull the ovaries and fallopian tubes toward the midline, a finding known as the 'kissing ovary' sign, or to encase the ovary, resulting in an appearance similar to that of a complex cystic solid mass. Predictably pyosalpinx and hematosalpinx have similar imaging characteristics, such as adhesions and the kissing ovary sign. MRI is the most useful modality to differentiate between the two, as imaging findings are more specific and allow better characterisation of blood products.

Reference

Moyle PL, Kataoka MY, Nakai A, *et al.* Nonovarian cystic lesions of the pelvis. *Radiographics.* 2010; **30**(4): 921–38.

Case D

History

A 57-year-old male with painful, swollen ankles

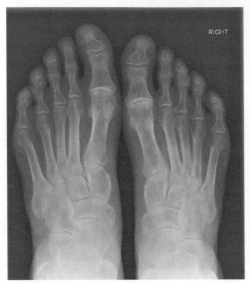

Figure i Feet radiograph

Figure ii Ankles radiograph

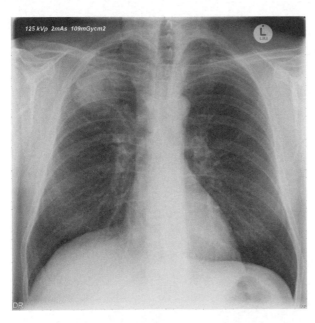

Figure iii Chest radiograph

Observations and interpretation

Feet radiograph:
- uniform periosteal reaction along the second, third and fourth metatarsals bilaterally;
- no focal lytic lesions are demonstrated.

Ankles radiograph:
- uniform periosteal reaction seen at the medial right distal fibula and anterior distal tibia;
- the left ankle (single lateral projection) has a normal appearance.

Chest radiograph:
- large rounded soft tissue density mass within the left upper zone, which is suspicious for a primary malignancy;
- no associated rib destruction or evidence of hilar enlargement;
- no further masses are seen;
- the heart size is within normal limits.

Main diagnosis

Appearances are in keeping with hypertrophic pulmonary osteoarthropathy secondary to a presumed primary lung malignancy.

Differential diagnoses

There are a number of other causes for the periosteal reaction, including acromegaly, thyroid acropachy, venous stasis and fibrous dysplasia, but these are all less likely.

Further management

Urgent referral to a chest physician for further assessment, including staging CT chest, percutaneous biopsy and discussion at Lung MDT meeting

Discussion

Hypertrophic pulmonary osteoarthropathy presents clinically with arthralgia and painful, swollen joints. The aetiology is unknown. The main feature radiographically, is of symmetric diaphyseal and metaphyseal periosteal new bone formation.

Hypertrophic osteoarthropathy can be primary or secondary. The primary form is usually familial, more common in males, developing in adolescence. It is also known as pachydermoperiostitis, a spectrum ranging from periostitis alone to a more severe form that involves periostitis, clubbed digits and skin thickening. Differentials for this appearance include thyroid acropachy, occurring after surgical resection of the thyroid gland for hyperthyroidism, as well as vascular insufficiency.

Secondary hypertrophic osteoarthropathy is a painful periostitis that affects the extremities and is associated with several disease processes, particularly bronchial carcinoma. It also occurs with other respiratory conditions (pleural fibroma, chronic suppurative diseases, cyanotic heart disease), gastrointestinal diseases (biliary cirrhosis, inflammatory bowel disease) and others. The appearances on bone scintigraphy have been described as the 'double stripe' sign, reflecting symmetrically increased uptake along the cortical margins of the diaphysis of long, tubular bones. The characteristic appearances generally regress on both radiographs and bone scintigraphy after treatment of the underlying cause.

Reference
Manaster BJ, May DA, Disler DG. *Musculoskeletal Radiology: the requisites*. 3rd ed. Philadelphia, USA. Mosby; 2007.

Case E

History

83-year-old female, previous history of breast carcinoma, on herceptin and bisphosphonates

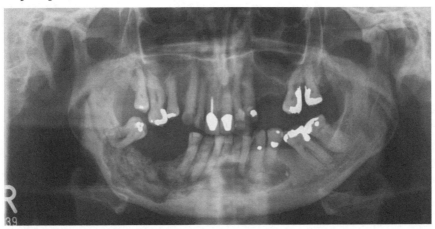

Figure i Orthopantomogram

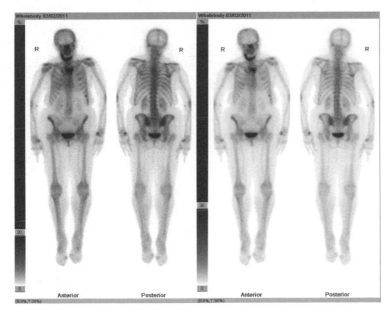

Figure ii Bone scan

Observations and interpretation

Orthopantomogram:

- area of mixed sclerosis and lucency seen within the right side of the mandible;
- diffuse sclerosis extending towards the midline and laterally within the mandible;
- no evidence of periosteal reaction, associated soft tissue mass or cortical breach.

Bone scan:

- intense uptake seen within the right side of mandible;
- uptake at the sternoclavicular joints bilaterally is most likely to be due to degenerative change, in view of the patient's age.

Main diagnosis

Osteonecrosis of the mandible, in view of the history of bisphosphonate use and diffuse sclerosis

Differential diagnoses

- Metastatic involvement of the mandible, with the predominantly sclerotic appearances on plain film, correlating with the osteoblastic bone scan appearances and the expected appearance of breast secondaries
- Primary bone neoplasm of the mandible, such as osteosarcoma, although less likely, as multifocal lucencies within the mandible and no periosteal reaction

Further management

Refer to Head and Neck/Maxillofacial MDT meeting

Discussion

Bisphosphonates are used in the treatment of osteoporosis, Paget's disease, pain from osseous metastases and malignancy-related hypercalcaemia. Bisphosphonates have a mechanism of action of decreasing bone turnover by inhibiting osteoclast-mediated bone resorption. The clinical presentation in these patients is of poorly healing extraction sockets and painful bone exposure. Biopsy is avoided where possible to avoid poor healing after intervention, unless there is a strong suspicion of metastases. Therefore, imaging may be employed more frequently to confirm the diagnosis. It is important to note that bisphosphonates persist in the skeletal system for up to 10 years and therefore complications may occur even after therapy has stopped.

Most commonly, osseous sclerosis is seen radiographically. The alveolar crest is a small area of cortical bone of the mandible in between each tooth and the bone density of the mandible is equal throughout the bone. Early changes with bisphosphonates include thickening of the alveolar crest and sclerosis at this area. Sequential imaging shows diffuse sclerotic involvement of the mandible. Reactive sclerosis tends to be localised around inflammatory foci, rather than diffuse. Less frequently seen appearances, and more commonly associated with infection, include osteolysis, soft tissue swelling, periosteal new bone formation and periapical lucencies.

Other lesions that occur in the mandible include ameloblastoma (locally aggressive, multiloculated, lytic lesion with solid component), osteosarcoma/Ewing's sarcoma (dense hyperostotic process or lytic mass, with periosteal reaction), metastases (commonly from renal, breast, lung or thyroid in adults, neuroblastoma in children) and lymphoma (usually non-Hodgkin's lymphoma, permative process).

References

Phal PM, Myall RW, Assael LA, *et al.* Imaging findings of bisphosphonate-associated osteonecrosis of the jaws. *AJNR Am J Neuroradiol.* 2007; **28**(6): 1139–45.

Grossman RI, Yousem DM. *Neuroradiology: the requisites.* 2nd ed. Philadelphia, USA: Mosby; 2003.

Case F

History

A 12-year-old female with cough

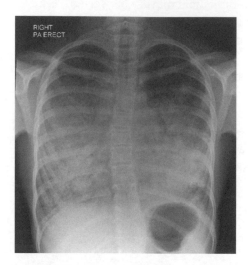

Figure i Chest radiograph

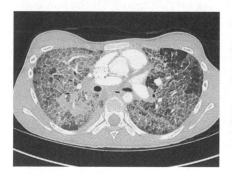

Figure ii Arterial phase CT of the chest (lung windows)

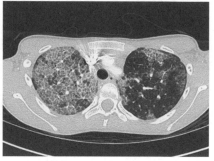

Figure iii Arterial phase CT of the chest (lung windows)

Observations and interpretation

Chest radiograph:

- widespread airspace opacification in the mid and lower zones, with the apices spared;
- the heart size is within normal limits.

CT of the chest (arterial phase):
- diffuse bilateral ground-glass opacification with septal thickening in the mid and lower zones;
- consolidation is noted in the apical segment of the right upper lobe;
- normal vasculature and venous drainage;
- no mediastinal lymphadenopathy.

Main diagnosis
Multifocal areas of ground-glass opacification with septal thickening, of which extrinsic allergic alveolitis, drug reaction or pulmonary alveolar proteinosis would be potential causes

Differential diagnoses
See 'Main diagnosis'

Further management
- Referral to the chest physicians and cardiothoracic surgeons
- For consideration of open lung biopsy

Discussion
The underlying cause in this case was found to be pulmonary alveolar proteinosis (PAP). PAP occurs from filling of the alveoli with proteinaeous, lipid-rich material that is positive on Periodic acid–Schiff (PAS) staining. There is an associated inflammatory response in the adjacent interstitium. It is thought to be due to an abnormality of surfactant production, metabolism or clearance by type II alveolar cells and macrophages. The subtypes are congenital, idiopathic and secondary. Most cases are idiopathic but it can also occur secondary to exposure from silica, or in association with haematological disorders, such as lymphoma or leukaemia. The congenital form is not universally accepted as a separate subtype and may represent 'chronic pneumonitis of infancy', which has a poor prognosis overall.

The clinical presentation is variable and can range from mild progressive dyspnea to respiratory failure. In adults, there is a strong association with smoking. The lactate dehydrogenase level is the most commonly elevated serological marker but is still a non-specific finding. Blood gases show a hypoxic picture with reduced gas exchange on spirometry. Definite diagnosis is made by open lung biopsy or bronchoalveolar lavage. The bronchial washings contain intraalveolar deposits of proteinaceous material, dissolved cholesterol and eosinophilic globules. Treatment includes whole-lung lavage, which may need to be repeated several times.

The chest radiograph typically shows bilateral, central and symmetric lung opacities, with sparing of the apices and costophrenic angles. The opacities may have a range of appearances, such as ground glass with indistinct margins, reticular or reticulonodular, or consolidation with air bronchograms. Appearances are similar to those of pulmonary interstitial oedema without the associated features of pulmonary oedema (pleural effusions and cardiomegaly).

Chest CT gives improved anatomic detail and reflects disease extent. The main feature is of a 'crazy paving' pattern, with smoothly thickened septal lines superimposed on areas of ground-glass opacity. These abnormal areas typically have a geographical pattern with sharp margins.

The crazy paving sign is seen on CT and is a reticular pattern superimposed on ground-glass opacity. The underlying abnormalities involve both the airspace and the interstitium. The reticular opacities may represent interlobular septal thickening, thickening of the intralobular interstitium, irregular areas of fibrosis. As well as PAP, the crazy paving sign is also seen with *Pneumocystic carinii* pneumonia, bronchoalveolar carcinoma, sarcoidosis, lipoid pneumonia, adult respiratory distress or pulmonary haemorrhage. The differential can often be narrowed down by the presence of additional radiological findings, the history and the clinical signs.

References

Lee CH. The crazy-paving sign. *Radiology*. 2007; **243**(3): 905–6.

Frazier AA, Franks TJ, Cooke EO, *et al*. From the archives of the AFIP: pulmonary alveolar proteinosis. *Radiographics*. 2008; **28**(3): 883–99.

Paper 3

Case A
History
A 6-year-old girl with a new limp and no previous medical history

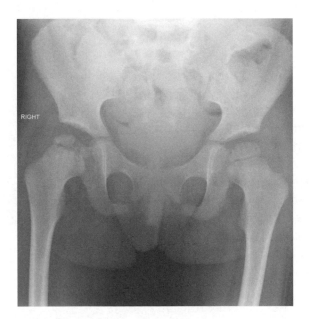

Figure i Radiograph of the pelvis

Observations and interpretation
Radiograph of the pelvis (anteroposterior):
- minor widening of the right femoral-acetabular joint space;
- loss of height of the right femoral capital epiphysis; it is also irregular and fragmented;

- local increased bone density;
- no right acetabular modeling abnormality;
- the left hip appears unremarkable, as does the rest of the bony pelvis.

Main diagnosis
Perthes' disease

Differential diagnoses
Other causes of avascular necrosis – for example, steroid use, trauma or sickle-cell anaemia. These risk factors should be apparent from the clinical history.

Further management
- Referral to orthopaedic surgeons for appropriate management
- 'Frog-leg view' radiograph to look for subtle Perthes' of the contralateral hip

Discussion
Perthes' disease (or Legg-Calvé-Perthes disease) is idiopathic avascular necrosis of the femoral head in the paediatric population. This condition is more common in males and usually occurs between the ages of 4 and 8 years. It is commonly unilateral but is bilateral in up to 15% of cases. It is important to diagnose Perthes' as early as possible, as orthopaedic management can limit the long-term sequelae. The principles of management are to maintain acetabular coverage and prevent lateral subluxation; this can be done conservatively with abduction bracing or surgically via osteotomy.

Radiographically, there are a number of findings that indicate this diagnosis and can be broadly categorised into early, intermediate and late.
- Early signs include a widened joint space, which is usually due to an effusion, and sclerosis and subchondral fissure fractures, which are best seen on frog-leg views.
- In more progressive disease or intermediate phase, there is fragmentation of the epiphysis, lateralisation of ossification, occasionally cyst formation and bone demineralisation, usually occurring in the femoral neck.
- The latter stages are characterised by a flattened, distorted femoral head, modeling deformities such as coxa magna and plana and eventually signs of secondary osteoarthritis.

In the early stages, changes may be absent or extremely subtle on plain film.

MRI can be utilised to detect early disease or in cases of diagnostic uncertainty. MRI is extremely sensitive and can often show avascular necrosis where plain films or radionuclide studies are normal. MRI can also be useful to help plan treatment, for example, evaluation of acetabular coverage.

Reference
Saini A, Saifuddin A. MRI of osteonecrosis. *Clin Radiol.* 2004; **59**(12): 1079–93.

Case B

History

A 74-year-old female with increasing abdominal pain and distension

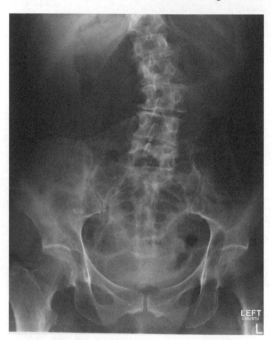

Figure i Abdominal radiograph

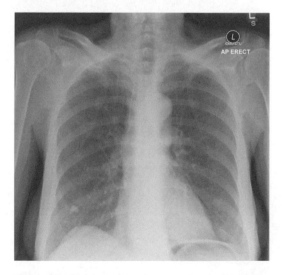

Figure ii Chest radiograph

Observations and interpretation
Abdominal radiograph:
- evidence of intramural air in multiple segments of bowel – this appears to be mainly colon;
- evidence of pneumoperitoneum;
- in the right upper quadrant there is gas in a branching pattern most consistent with gas in the portal venous system.

Chest radiograph:
- free air under the hemidiaphragms;
- the lungs are clear bar calcified granulomas;
- normal cardiomediastinum.

Main diagnosis
Ischaemic colitis with perforation and gas in the portal vein

Differential diagnoses
Other causes of perforation include diverticular disease, peptic ulcer disease, inflammatory bowel disease and appendicitis. The causes of pneumotosis are manifold, including acute and non-acute pathology.

Further management
- Urgent referral to general/on-call surgical team.
- A CT of the abdomen and pelvis may be indicated.

Discussion
Pneumotosis coli is defined as gas within the bowel wall. CT sensitivity is much greater than plain films in detecting this; occasionally it can be difficult to differentiate gas in the periphery of lumen from true intramural air.

This is an interesting phenomenon, as the causes range from benign where it can be an incidental finding to evidence of significant life-threatening pathology.

Fifteen per cent of cases are idiopathic and usually involve the colon. It can be associated with pulmonary disease (asthma, emphysema and positive end-expiratory pressures) and a wide variety of bowel pathology from inflammatory bowel disease to adynamic ileus. It can be iatrogenic, it can be related to medication – particularly steroids and chemotherapy agents – and it is associated with graft-versus-host disease. Serious life-threatening pathologies that are indicated by pneumatosis include intestinal ischaemia, obstruction, enteritis, toxic megacolon and trauma.

Gas in the portal venous system is an important finding. The most serious and most frequent cause of portomesenteric vein gas in adults is mesenteric ischaemia. However, the association of portomesenteric vein gas with this disease process does not imply a worse prognosis; thus, surgical treatment should not be excluded when this sign is present. Several other disease processes have been described recently as causes of portomesenteric vein gas. In the majority of cases, particularly when portomesenteric vein gas is secondary to invasive procedures, surgery is not required and the prognosis is favourable. Findings of portomesenteric vein gas at CT should be carefully evaluated in the context of clinical findings before making decisions regarding diagnosis and therapy. On the basis of our experience and descriptions in the literature, we have divided these causes into four groups: (1) intestinal wall alterations (inflammatory bowel disease, mesenteric ischaemia), (2) bowel distention (gastric and bowel dilatation due to spontaneous, traumatic and iatrogenic causes), (3) intra-abdominal sepsis (e.g. diverticulitis, abdominal wall gangrene, pylophlebitis), and (4) unknown causes (transplantation, pneumatosis intestinalis, corticosteroid therapy, chronic pulmonary disease).

(There are many causes of pneumoperitoneum. The most common aetiologies of spontaneous pneumoperitoneum are peptic ulcer perforation, ischaemia, bowel obstruction, inflammation including appendicitis and toxic megacolon.)

In this case, perforation secondary to malignant obstruction would probably be the most likely cause, although the primary lesion is not definitively visualised, as there is evidence of obstruction with bowel dilatation and pneumotosis, luminal perforation and metastatic disease (adrenal metastasis).

References

Rha SE, Ha HK, Lee S-H, *et al*. CT and MR imaging findings of bowel ischemia from various primary causes. *Radiographics*. 2000; **20**(1): 29–42.

Sebastià C, Quiroga S, Espin E, *et al*. Portomesenteric vein gas: pathologic mechanisms, CT findings, and prognosis. *Radiographics*. 2000; **20**(5): 1213–24.

Urban BA, Fishman EK. Tailored helical CT evaluation of acute abdomen. *Radiographics*. 2000; **20**(3): 725–49.

Case C

History
A 44-year-old male presents with haematuria and loin pain

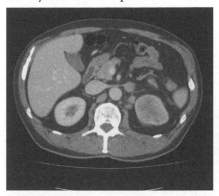

Figure i Portal venous phase CT of the abdomen

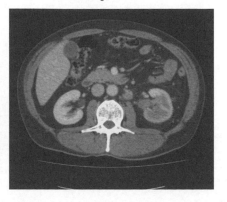

Figure ii Portal venous phase CT of the abdomen

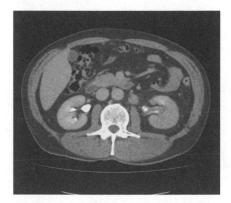

Figure iii Delayed phase CT of the abdomen

Observations and interpretation
CT of the abdomen and pelvis (portal venous and delayed phase):
- an infiltrating ill-defined mass has replaced the upper pole and most of the interpolar region of the left kidney – this is suspicious for a malignant process;
- involvement of the upper pole infundibulum and renal sinus fat;
- minimal enhancement and no excretion is seen in the left upper pole and there is a filling defect within the renal pelvis – this could be either tumour or clot;

- stranding in the perinephric fat with no evidence of direct spread beyond;
- the left renal vein and inferior vena cava look satisfactory;
- multiple enlarged left para-aortic nodes;
- the left ureter is not fully opacified but there are no features of distal involvement;
- gas is noted in the urinary bladder but this looks otherwise normal, as does the rest of the renal tract;
- likely simple liver cyst; the rest of the solid organs are unremarkable.

Main diagnosis

Infiltrating transitional cell carcinoma (TCC) with likely para-aortic nodal involvement but no definite distant metastatic disease

Differential diagnoses

- Other malignant process: renal cell carcinoma, metastases to kidney or even lymphoma (very unlikely, as usually bilateral and gives rise to enlarged smooth kidneys)
- Inflammatory/infective process – it would be hard to explain the filling defects in the collecting system, but these may be due to clot.

Further management

- Referral to the Urological MDT meeting
- Discuss obtaining tissue –the urologists could do this with a retrograde ureteroscopy; percutaneous approach is not favoured in potential transitional cell carcinoma, as there is a theoretical risk of seeding
- CT of the chest to complete staging
- Consider ultrasound, MRI or interval CT imaging of the liver to follow up the low-density lesions

Discussion

TCC can occur anywhere in the renal tract where there is transitional epithelium. TCC of the upper urinary tract is a common malignancy affecting the genitourinary tract. It is commonly multifocal, with a high incidence of recurrence requiring rigorous urothelial surveillance; in fact, the hallmark of TCC is multiplicity and recurrence. It is usually a papillary-type lesion with a frond-like structure. A more aggressive form is infiltrating disease but fortunately this is less common.

Diagnosis of upper tract TCC is heavily dependent on imaging. Understanding the appearances of upper tract TCC on different imaging techniques is important in the accurate interpretation of imaging studies.

CT urography is very useful at assessing these types of lesions although there can be a tendency to over stage. Typical appearances include filling defects on the excretory phase, mass in the renal pelvis, infiltration of the adjacent renal parenchyma and variable tumour enhancement. US is often used as a first-line investigation in someone with haematuria, but it can be difficult to detect this tumour with this modality; even the larger masses can be difficult to appreciate, as they are usually of low reflectivity and central in position. Therefore, indirect signs on US such as the obliteration of fat planes within the renal pelvis and calyceal dilatation are obviously important to recognise.

TNM staging of upper urinary tract transitional cell carcinoma

TNM	Disease extent
Ta	Noninvasive papillary carcinoma that is confined to urothelium and projecting toward the lumen
Tis	Carcinoma in situ: flat tumour with high-grade histologic features that is confined to urothelium
T1	Tumour invades subepithelial connective tissue (lamina propria)
T2	Tumour invades muscularis
T3	Renal pelvis: tumour invades beyond the muscularis into the peripelvic fat or renal parenchyma
	Ureter: tumour invades beyond the muscularis into the periureteric fat
T4	Tumour invades adjacent organs, the pelvic or abdominal wall, or through the kidney into the perinephric fat
N0	No regional lymph node metastases
N1	Metastasis to a single lymph node that is <2 cm in greatest dimension
N2	Metastasis to a single lymph node that is 2–5 cm in greatest dimension or to multiple lymph nodes, none of which is >5 cm in greatest dimension
N3	Metastasis to a lymph node that is >5 cm in greatest dimension
M0	No distant metastasis
M1	Distant metastases

References
Anderson EM, Murphy R, Rennie AT, *et al.* Multidetector computed tomography urography (MDCTU) for diagnosing urothelial malignancy. *Clin Radiol.* 2007; **62**(4): 324–32.

Vikram R, Sandler CM, Ng CS. Imaging and staging of transitional cell carcinoma: part 2, upper urinary tract. *AJR Am J Roentgenol.* 2009; **192**(6): 1488–93.

Case D

History

A 22-year-old female with a 4-week history of swelling of the right knee

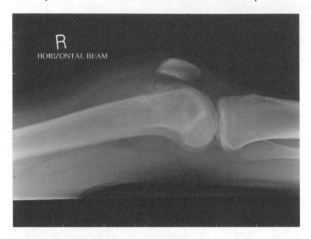

Figure i radiograph of the knee (lateral)

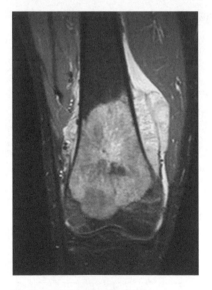

Figure ii Sagittal T1 MRI

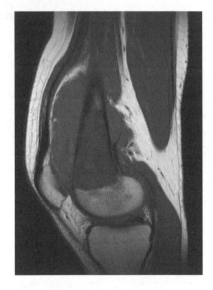

Figure iii Coronal STIR MRI

Observations and interpretation

radiograph of the right knee:
- soft tissue swelling with distortion of the fat planes;
- calcification is seen in the soft tissues of the suprapatellar pouch.

MRI of the right knee (knee: T1 sagittal, coronal STIR, axial proton density: whole leg: T1 axial):
- abnormal low signal in the distal femur and extending into the adjacent soft tissues, where there is a heterogeneous soft tissue mass;
- the low signal contacts the intercondylar notch but does not cross the joint;
- periosteal elevation is present;
- no evidence of skip lesions.

Main diagnosis

Primary osteosarcoma

Differential diagnoses

Lymphoma

Further management

- Complete staging imaging with MRI of the whole femur, hip and knee
- CT of the chest for further staging
- Referral to bone tumour unit for multidisciplinary discussion and further management plan

Discussion

Osteosarcoma is a common primary malignant bone tumour. It produces osteoid matrix and hence is often detectable on plain radiographs. The World Health Organization has classified osteosarcoma into eight subtypes: (1) conventional, (2) telangiectatic, (3) small cell, (4) low-grade central, (5) secondary, (6) parosteal, (7) periosteal and (8) high-grade surface. Imaging plays an important role in the diagnosis and management of these patients, for initial staging, biopsy planning and follow up.

The conventional subtype is the most common subtype, particularly seen in children and adolescents. In adults, it can arise *de novo* or it can be associated with a pre-existing abnormality such as Paget's disease or previous radiotherapy. It is identified on plain radiographs as an intramedullary mass with cloud-like bone formation in the metaphyses of long bones. MRI appearances include low-signal primary lesion, with extra-osseous soft tissue mass. It is important to note any disease on the other side of adjacent joints and also the presence of skip lesions within the same bone, as this affects management and prognosis.

Tumour staging is by the American Joint Committee on Cancer staging system of TMN staging. The T stage involves the size and extent of the tumour: T1 if smaller than 8 cm, T2 if larger than 8 cm, T3 if skip metastases are detected. Smaller tumours generally have a better prognosis and skip lesions, in a high-grade tumour, a poor prognosis. The nodal stage describes either absent local nodes (N0), presence of regional nodes (N1) or not assessed (NX). M0 indicates there are no detected metastases; M1 indicates if regional or distant metastases (M1a describes lung-only metastases; M1b involves other distant sites). Lung-only metastases, particularly if solitary, have a better prognosis than other distant disease.

MRI is the optimal modality for assessment of tumour size and presence of skip metastases (T1 or STIR sagittal or coronal sequences preferred). Post-gadolinium imaging can be helpful to determine sites of necrosis and viable tumour for biopsy planning. Skeletal scintigraphy with an osteosarcoma primary is sometimes recommended to assess for bone metastases elsewhere.

References

Stacy GS, Mahal RS, Peabody TD. Staging of bone tumors: a review with illustrative examples. *AJR Am J Roentgenol.* 2006; **186**(4): 967–76.

Yarmish G, Klein MJ, Landa J, *et al.* Imaging characteristics of primary osteosarcoma: nonconventional subtypes. *Radiographics.* 2010; **30**(6): 1653–72.

Case E

History

A 53-year-old male with abnormal hormone levels

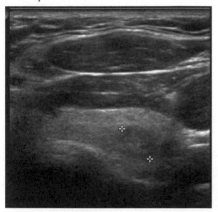

Figure i US of the neck – left thyroid lobe, transverse section

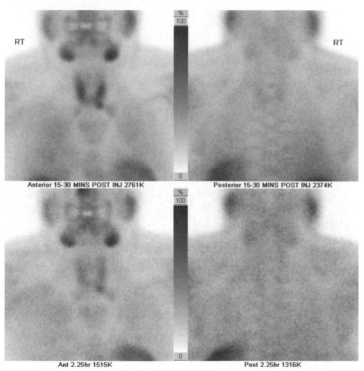

Figure ii Single-photon emission CT parathyroid scan

Observations and interpretation

Ultrasound of neck/parathyroids:
- there is a low echogenicity area seen at the lower pole of the thyroid (on the left);
- there is evidence of posterior acoustic enhancement;
- in the appropriate clinical context, appearances are consistent with a parathyroid adenoma.

Nuclear medicine parathyroid scan with single-photon emission CT (SPECT):
- uniform uptake by the thyroid;
- at the lower pole of the left thyroid lobe, there is a discrete focus of tracer uptake, seen at 15–30 minutes post injection and slightly less intensely at 2.25 hours post injection;
- this is in the region of the parathyroid, and would be in keeping with a parathyroid adenoma;
- no evidence of uptake seen within the chest or mediastinum.

Main diagnosis

In view of the functional and ultrasound findings, parathyroid adenoma is the most likely diagnosis.

Differential diagnoses
- A thyroid adenoma can be a false positive.
- Hyperplasia is unlikely to affect a single parathyroid gland.
- Parathyroid carcinoma can also be hyperfunctioning but it is rare relative to adenoma.

Further management

Referral to Head and Neck surgery for removal of adenoma

Discussion

Parathyroid adenoma is suspected clinically in patients with hypercalcemia and raised parathyroid hormone levels (primary hyperparathyroidism). There is a variety of imaging modalities that can be used for investigation of hyperparathyroidism, with nuclear medicine studies having approximately 90% sensitivity, CT 75%, ultrasound 60% and MRI 70%.

Nuclear medicine investigation of hyperparathyroidism is highly sensitive for adenomas larger than 300 mg in size (85%–90%). The technique involves intravenous injection of technitium-99m sestamibi followed by two phases of planar imaging, first at 10 minutes, followed by later imaging, at 2 hours. This is known as the washout method, as it is possible to assess the differential wash out from thyroid tissue and hyperfunctioning parathyroid tissue. It is important to image the chest, as ectopic parathyroid tissue may be found in the anterior mediastinum, thyroid, thymus, parapharyngeal region chest and lower neck. Parathyroid adenomas may even be found within the thyroid. Initial images show prominent thyroid uptake, with focal uptake seen in parathyroid adenomas. On delayed imaging, most of the thyroid uptake has washed out, leaving any adenomas or hyperfunctioning parathyroid tissue as a focus of residual activity with a high target-to-background ratio. Another method involves two isotopes, iodine-123 and technitium-99m sestamibi, and permits subtraction as the iodine-123 is taken up by both thyroid and parathyroid tissue. For localisation in some cases, SPECT, or even SPECT combined with CT, can be useful.

Ultrasound can be used to localise parathyroid adenomas that have been identified on functional imaging. Sonographic appearances are of a slightly triangular or round hypoechoic lesion, usually posterior to the lower poles of the thyroid. Normal parathyroids are generally not identified on ultrasound.

MRI can be helpful in identifying adenomas within the mediastinum. Typical appearances are of high signal on T2, low T1 signal with avid enhancement post contrast. However, up to 30% of adenomas have atypical features, such as high signal on T1 or intermediate T2 signal, reflecting cellular degeneration, intratumoural haemorrhage, fibrosis and haemosiderin deposition. Another pitfall with MRI is that lymph nodes and intrathyroid nodules can also be bright on T2. Therefore, the combination of cross-sectional and functional imaging is helpful to guide the clinician to potential adenomas in the more difficult cases.

References

Grossman RI, Yousem DM. *Neuroradiology: the requisites.* 2nd ed. Philadelphia, USA. Mosby; 2003.

Ziessman HA, O'Malley JP, Thrall JH. *Nuclear Medicine: the requisites.* 3rd ed. Philadelphia, USA. Mosby; 2006.

Case F

History

An 82-year-old male patient with dyspnoea

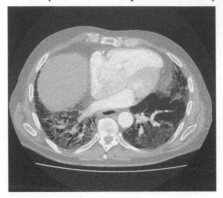 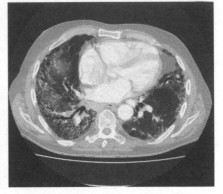

Figure i Arterial phase CT of the chest (lung windows)

Figure ii Arterial phase CT of the chest (lung windows)

Observations and interpretation

CT of the chest (arterial phase):

- peripheral honeycomb pattern with bronchiolectasis, predominantly at the bases but also in the anterior aspect of the upper lobes;
- volume loss of the right hemithorax with deviation of the trachea to the right, secondary to right apical fibrosis;
- no focal lung lesion or endobronchial mass;
- no significant lymphadenopathy;
- evidence of previous cholecystectomy, with pneumobilia, presumably due to previous endoscopic retrograde cholangiopancreatography;
- no bone lesions.

Main diagnosis
Usual interstitial pneumonitis (UIP)

Differential diagnoses
Non-specific interstitial pneumonitis, due to the involvement of the upper lobes

Further management
Referral to a respiratory physician for further management

Discussion
UIP is the most common of the idiopathic interstitial pneumonias, and is also known as idiopathic pulmonary fibrosis. The pathological process is of inflammation, which can lead to pulmonary fibrosis. This group of processes includes UIP, acute interstitial pneumonia, non-specific interstitial pneumonia, cryptogenic organising pneumonia, desquamative interstitial pneumonia (DIP), lymphoid interstitial pneumonia and respiratory bronchiolitis–associated interstitial lung disease.

The abnormalities seen in UIP represent a spectrum of the underlying pathological processes, with early features of macrophage proliferation in the alveolar space and minor, uniform interstitial thickening, with later fibrosis and ongoing interstitial thickening. The patient demographic is typically male in the fifth to seventh decades of life. UIP is usually idiopathic, but in a third of cases it is associated with collagen vascular disorders, such as rheumatoid arthritis. Early radiographic appearances are of fine reticular or ground-glass opacities, progressing to a coarse reticular or reticulonodular pattern, and followed by honeycomb cysts (3–10 mm in diameter) and progressive volume loss. If extensive, there may be associated pulmonary arterial hypertension. The typical location of these changes is in the peripheral and basal parts of the lungs, which may differentiate from other interstitial processes. Mildly enlarged mediastinal nodes are associated. The mean survival is poor, with an average of 5 years, because of complications of respiratory or cardiac failure, as well as the increased risk of malignancy – particularly adenocarcinoma.

Acute interstitial pneumonia is an acute, aggressive idiopathic interstitial pneumonia and is sometimes referred to as idiopathic acute respiratory distress syndrome. Radiographic features include diffuse ground-glass opacity, air bronchograms, with fibrosis developing less commonly than in UIP. Mortality occurs in over two-thirds of those affected.

Cryptogenic organising pneumonia is caused by the widespread deposition of granulation tissue within peribronchiolar airspaces and is often

61

associated with a long history of subacute infection. Features on high-resolution CT include patchy ground-glass opacities, with a subpleural or peribronchial distribution, with bronchiectasis and bronchial wall thickening. This condition usually responds well to corticosteroid therapy and has a better prognosis than UIP.

Respiratory bronchiolitis–associated interstitial lung disease is only seen in smokers and is due to inflammation around and within the bronchioles. Radiographic appearances can be normal; however, on high-resolution CT, ground-glass opacities and centrilobular nodules may be seen with an upper lobe distribution. There is some overlap with DIP.

DIP is also seen predominantly in smokers, and in younger patients than UIP, but it may be difficult to distinguish between DIP and UIP on imaging alone. DIP is characterised by bibasal reticular opacities, with ground-glass opacities seen less commonly and honeycombing a rare feature. However, DIP responds better to steroids and has a better prognosis than UIP.

Lymphoid interstitial pneumonia is seen more commonly in women and is characterised by ground-glass opacities, perivascular cysts, septal thickening and centrilobular nodules. It also has a basilar predominance.

Non-specific interstitial pneumonia describes any condition that does not fit into one of the other categories. It is often associated with collagen vascular disorders or drug reactions, and there are cellular and fibrotic subtypes.

Classifying these processes (which may sometimes require a surgical lung biopsy) can assist with treatment and prognosis.

Reference

Mueller-Mang C, Grosse C, Schmid K, *et al.* What every radiologist should know about idiopathic interstitial pneumonias. *Radiographics.* 2007; **27**(3): 595–615.

Paper 4

Case A
History
An 11-month-old girl admitted with urinary retention; pelvic mass on examination

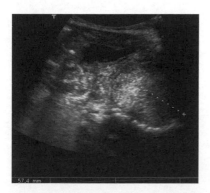

Figure i Transabdominal pelvic ultrasound

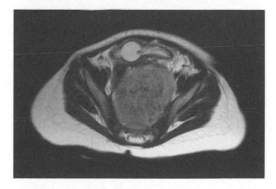

Figure ii Axial proton density MRI

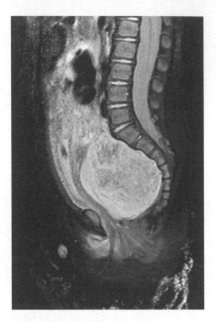

Figure iii Sagittal STIR MRI

Observations and interpretation

Transabdominal pelvic ultrasound:
- large presacral mass;
- mass is of heterogeneous echogenicity consistent with soft tissue.

Pelvic MRI (axial proton density and sagittal STIR):
- large presacral soft tissue mass;
- mass returns slightly heterogeneous signal, being predominantly isointense with muscle on T1 weighting and of high signal on T2 weighting;
- best seen on the coronal sequence, the mass contains one or two foci of high signal most likely to correspond to fluid, suggesting a degree of tumour necrosis;
- no definite evidence of fat or calcification within the mass;
- closely apposed to the sacrum but no evidence of destruction;
- mass is displacing and compressing the recto sigmoid to the right of the pelvic cavity and is displacing the bladder supero-anteriorly;
- left external iliac vessels are draped over the dome of the mass but there is no evidence of a large median sacral artery;
- no lymphadenopathy or further masses seen;
- no congenital spinal abnormality.

Main diagnosis
Sacrococcygeal teratoma

Differential diagnoses
- Rhabdomyosarcoma arises from the anterior wall of the vagina in girls and the prostate or bladder in boys. It is usually possible on MRI to distinguish this point of origin to differentiate from a sacrococcygeal teratoma.
- Neuroblastoma: this is rare and is characterised radiologically by amorphous irregular calcification.
- Sacral chordoma: this is a rare tumour that originates from the remnants of the primitive notocord. It is often associated with destruction of the sacrum and flocculated calcification.
- Other paediatric sacral masses include anterior sacral meningoceles or myelomeningoceles, neuroenteric cysts, ependymomas and haemangiomas. However, the imaging features of these lesions are unlike those in this case.

Further management
- Referral to Paediatric surgeons and discussion at MDT meeting
- Consider radiologically guided biopsy of the lesion

Discussion
The presacral or retrorectal space is located between the rectum and the sacrococcygeal part of the spine. In embryologic development, the remodelling and regression of the neuroectoderm, notochord, hindgut, and proctoderm help to define this space. The presacral space contains a variety of tissues, including fat, mesenchymal tissue, lymph nodes, nerve plexuses, and vessels. Hence, a variety of tumoural lesions may affect this area.

Sacrococcygeal teratomas are the most common tumour in newborns, nearly three quarters present in the first few days of life. There is also a slight female predilection. The histopathology ranges from benign to malignant; the risk of malignancy is associated with age – at more than 2 months there is an up to 90% probability of malignancy.

These tumours are associated with other congenital anomalies in up to 20% of cases. These include the Currarino triad, also known as ASP triad (anorectal malformation, sacrococcygeal osseous defect, and presacral mass), spinal dysraphism, sacral agenesis, dislocation of the hip, and renal and gastrointestinal anomalies. Prenatal complications include polyhydramnios and haemorrhage, which can lead to foetal hydrops.

These tumours are often large and cause deformity of the sacrococcyx. Radiological characteristics include calcification, amorphous or formed (such as teeth), and cystic components. On ultrasound, the lesion is usually mixed solid and cystic, and demonstrates marked vascularity. On MRI, the tumour is predominantly heterogeneous on T1 sequences as a result of fat, soft tissue and calcification. Even if the tumour is on the malignant end of the spectrum, it frequently has a lobulated and well-defined margin.

Predominantly fatty or cystic lesions are usually benign, but conversely those containing haemorrhage or necrosis are more likely to be malignant.

Approximately 50% of benign teratomas contain calcification, whereas this feature is seldom observed in malignant tumours. Malignant teratomas may metastasize or extend into adjacent structures such as the spine or gluteal muscle. Such extension is also best depicted with MRI imaging.

Management is usually with surgical resection and, if malignant, chemotherapy.

Reference

Kocaoglu M, Frush DP. Pediatric presacral masses. *Radiographics.* 2006; **26**(3): 833–57.

Case B

History

A 58-year-old female with sudden-onset vomiting and abdominal distension

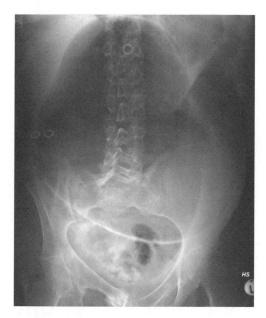

Figure i Abdominal radiograph

Observations and interpretation

Abdominal radiograph:

- grossly distended viscus in the central abdomen and left upper quadrant;
- otherwise, there is minimal bowel gas seen, a small amount is noted around the caecum and in the rectosigmoid;
- no evidence of pneumoperitoneum.

Main diagnosis
Gastric volvulus

Differential diagnoses
- Caecal or sigmoid volvulus – the lack of small or large bowel obstruction would be against this. Additionally, the position of the dilated viscus in the left upper quadrant favours a gastric volvulus.
- Gastric outlet obstruction from another cause – it would be unusual for the stomach to be so distended and gas filled.

Further management
- This is a surgical emergency – urgent discussion with the appropriate surgical team
- If clinically appropriate, consider CT for surgical planning/delineation of the volvulus

Discussion
The stomach is a relatively uncommon site of volvulus. Patients with acute gastric volvulus typically present with epigastric pain, nausea and vomiting. Borchardt's triad, a useful clinical triad for identifying gastric volvulus, consists of sudden epigastric pain, intractable retching, and inability to pass a nasogastric tube into the stomach.

A gastric volvulus is described as an abnormal degree of rotation of one part of the stomach around another part. Complete obstruction usually requires more than 180 degrees of rotation. As with other gastrointestinal volvuli, gastric volvulus is more prevalent in the elderly population, secondary to redundancy of the mesentery, which can then rotate around the mesenteric root. Further predisposing factors include eventration of the diaphragm, hiatus hernia, phrenic nerve paralysis and splenic abnormalities. Gastric volvulus is usually divided into two main subtypes: organoaxial and mesenteroaxial.

Organoaxial volvulus is more common, accounting for approximately two-thirds of cases. This is rotation around a line from cardia to pylorus – that is, the long axis of the stomach. It is most associated with large hiatus hernias and it results in a mirror-image stomach. The greater curvature becomes displaced superiorly and the lesser curvature is located more caudally in the abdomen. If the volvulus is severe or complete (twist greater than 180 degrees), gastric outlet obstruction occurs. Many patients have a less severe, incomplete or partial volvulus – a rotation of less than 180 degrees. In these cases, patients usually lack clinical symptoms of obstruction and exhibit no evidence of obstruction at imaging. In such cases, it is more accurate to describe the stomach as having an organoaxial position rather than an organoaxial volvulus, although an organoaxial position of the stomach predisposes it to future volvulus. It is unclear whether asymptomatic patients should be treated or followed up clinically. In general, the acuity and severity of symptoms dictate management.

Mesenteroaxial volvulus is rotation around an axis from the lesser to the greater curve (i.e the short axis), with resultant displacement of the antrum above the gastroesophageal junction. Fortunately, this is less common than organoaxial volvulus, as it is associated with more severe obstruction and disruption of vascular flow. Of note, appearances can become complex if there is a mixed organo and mesenteroaxial rotation.

Complications include gastric ischaemia and necrosis, gastric ulceration and peritonitis. Mortality is up to 80% in acute complete volvulus. Treatment is usually surgical via a gastropexy. CT is the most useful modality to investigate a potential volvulus as this can give information about obstruction, transition point and associated complications. Contrast studies may also be used to demonstrate the point of obstruction and orientation of the stomach.

Reference

Peterson CM, Anderson JS, Hara AK, *et al*. Volvulus of the gastrointestinal tract: appearances at multimodality imaging. *Radiographics*. 2009; **29**(5): 1281–93.

Case C

History

A 45-year-old woman with a palpable right breast lump

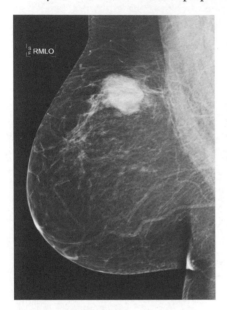

Figure i Radiograph – mammogram

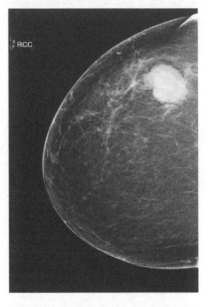

Figure ii Radiograph – mammogram

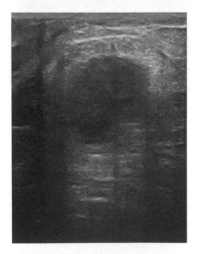

Figure iii Ultrasound of the right breast

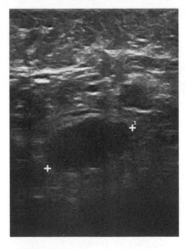

Figure iv Ultrasound of the right breast

Observations and interpretation
Radiograph – mammogram:
- the left breast appears normal;
- in the right breast there is an ill-defined 3.5 cm mass in the upper outer quadrant with some surrounding stromal thickening;
- large node in the right axilla.

Ultrasound of the right breast:
- there is an irregular low-reflectivity lesion in the upper outer quadrant;
- irregular node in the right axilla that has lost its fatty hilum.

Main diagnosis
Right breast cancer with right axillary nodal involvement; no distant metastases

Differential diagnoses
This lesion is malignant until proven otherwise. A benign process is unlikely, but an inflammatory lesion, for instance an abscess, could have these appearances.

Further management
- Urgent referral to the Breast MDT meeting and breast clinic
- Arrange targeted ultrasound of the lesion and core biopsies of the right breast lesion; consider fine needle aspiration or biopsy of the right axillary node
- Consider CT staging

Discussion
Breast cancer is the second most common cause of cancer-related death in women. Histopathologically there are numerous subtypes; the most common is invasive ductal carcinoma (approximately 65%), followed by invasive lobular carcinoma (approximately 15%), ductal carcinoma in situ (approximately 10%) and less frequent types such as tubular, medullary, mucinous and papillary carcinoma.

Mammogaphy is performed in two situations; as a screening tool or in symptomatic patients. The following characteristics are suggestive of a malignant process on mammography.
- Dominant mass seen on two tangential views.
- The border of the mass can be spiculated (for instance in invasive carcinomas), smooth (softer tumours such as medullary or mucinous

carcinoma) or lobulated (the likelihood of malignancy increases with the amount of lobulations).

- Asymmetric density.
- Microcalcification; fragmented, polymorphic, branching, granular.
- Architectural distortion.
- Diffuse increase in density.

Of note, there is a law referred to as Le Borgne's law that the greater the clinical size of the mass in comparison with the radiological size, the greater the probability of malignancy.

Ultrasound is a commonly used modality in characterising breast lesions and guiding biopsies. The appearances on ultrasound are discussed in more detail in Paper 11 Case C. CT is frequently used for staging disease in patients with moderate- to high-risk disease – for example, large masses and involved axillary nodes.

The most common site of metastases is the axillary lymph nodes. There are several features of nodes that suggest involvement. These include size (although this is not an absolute), loss of the normal fatty hilum, abnormal enhancement and irregularity. Of course if the nodes are clinically fixed this is also highly suspicious. Often, fine needle aspiration or biopsy of suspected axillary nodes is performed, as confirmed nodal disease affects management.

STAGING OF BREAST CANCER

TX: The tumour cannot be assessed

T0: No evidence of a tumour is present

Tis: The cancer may be lobular carcinoma in situ, ductal carcinoma in situ, or Paget's disease

T1: The tumour is 2 cm or smaller in diameter

T2: The tumour is 2–5 cm in diameter

T3: The tumour is more than 5 cm in diameter

T4: The tumour is any size, and it has attached itself to the chest wall and has spread to the pectoral (chest) lymph nodes

NX: Lymph nodes cannot be assessed (e.g. lymph nodes were previously removed)

N0: Cancer has not spread to lymph nodes

N1: Cancer has spread to the movable ipsilateral axillary lymph nodes

N2: Cancer has spread to ipsilateral lymph nodes, fixed to one another or to other structures under the arm

N3: Cancer has spread to the ipsilateral mammary lymph nodes or the ipsilateral supraclavicular lymph nodes

MX: Metastasis cannot be assessed

M0: No distant metastasis to other organs is present

M1: Distant metastasis to other organs has occurred

Case D

History
Unremitting left-sided sciatica

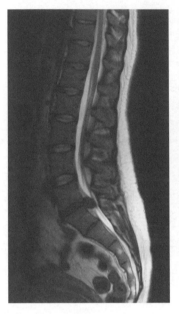 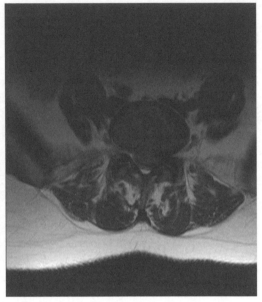

Figure i Sagittal T2 MRI   **Figure ii** Axial T2 MRI

Observations and interpretation
MRI of the lumbar spine (T1 and T2 sagittal, T1 and T2 axial):
- bone marrow signal is within normal limits;
- the conus lies at L1 and cord signal is normal;
- central/left paracentral large disc extrusion at the L5/S1 level that markedly narrows the spinal canal;
- the lateral recesses are narrowed bilaterally, with the left lateral recess obliterated; the descending S1 nerve roots, in particular those on the left, are compromised;
- the neural formamina are not affected;
- no evidence of annular tear or sequestered fragment.

Main diagnosis

Degenerative L5/S1 intervertebral disc extrusion with effacement of the left lateral recess

Differential diagnoses

No other differentials exist for this appearance

Further management

A spinal or neurosurgical surgical opinion is recommended for further management.

Discussion

Disc degeneration starts with tearing of the annulus fibrosis, concentric outer fibres first, followed by the inner radial fibres. Some of these annular tears are high signal on T2, called high-intensity zones, which represent neovascularity as well as rupture of the fibres. However, it is not clear whether the presence of an annular tear is also responsible for discogenic pain.

There is recognised terminology for the appearance of abnormal discs on MRI. A disc protrusion refers to a focal or broad-based smoothly marginated extension of the annulus beyond the vertebral margin, where the outer annulus/posterior longitudinal ligament complex is intact, or the base of the abnormal annular morphology is broader than the apex.

A disc extrusion has opposite appearances, where the outer annulus/posterior longitudinal ligament complex is clearly disrupted, or the base is narrower than the apex. A sequestration is a fragment of disc material that has broken off and is free in the epidural space.

Osseous changes may also be seen on either side of a degenerating or degenerated disc, which are referred to as Modic changes. The first change is of increased T2 endplate change and decreased T1 endplate change, which is due to inflammatory granulation tissue and oedema. Modic type 2 changes are of fatty change (low signal on T2 and high signal on T1), and Modic type 3 changes are thought to represent sclerosis and are low signal on T1- and T2-weighted images.

Reference

Helms CA. Lumbar spine: disk disease and stenosis. In: Brant WE, Helms CA. *Fundamentals of Diagnostic Radiology*. 3rd ed. Philadephia, USA: Lippincott, Williams & Wilkins; 2007. pp. 322–31.

Case E

History

A 39-year-old female with headache

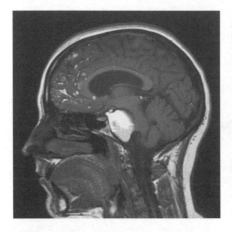

Figure i Sagittal T1 MRI

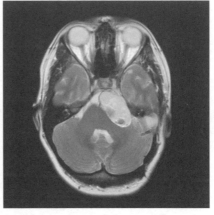

Figure ii Axial T2 MRI

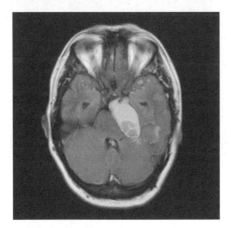

Figure iii Axial T1 MRI

Observations and interpretation
MRI of the head (sagittal T1, axial T2 and axial fluid-attenuated inversion recovery):

- heterogeneous signal mass at the left cerebellopontine angle, which is predominantly of high signal on fluid-attenuated inversion recovery, T1-, and T2-weighted sequences, in keeping with fat;
- some low-signal areas within the posterior-inferior aspect reflecting other tissue types;
- local mass effect on the pons, which is displaced posteriorly;
- the basilar artery runs along the anterior surface of the lesion;
- the configuration of the ventricles is preserved and the size is within normal limits;
- multiple high-signal locules within the subarachnoid space, in keeping with fat;
- the rest of the parenchyma and midline structures are normal.

Main diagnosis
Dermoid cyst at the left cerebellopontine angle with fat locules throughout the subarachnoid space

Differential diagnoses
None – this is an Aunt Minnie appearance

Further management
- Review of previous imaging
- Referral to neurosurgeons for further discussion and management

Discussion
It is helpful to use the location of a cyst to establish a differential diagnosis. It is helpful to assess whether a cyst is intra- or extra-axial, whether it is supra- or infratentorial, whether it is a midline lesion, whether it is intraparenchymal or intraventricular, whether it contains cerebrospinal fluid and if there are any distinguishing features such as calcification, enhancement or diffusion restriction.

Dermoid cysts are classified as congenital ectodermal inclusion cysts (as are epidermoid cysts). They are relatively rare (0.5% of primary intracranial tumours). They commonly occur in the midline, both supra and infratentorial, including in the sellar, parasellar, frontonasal regions, cerebellar vermis or within the fourth ventricle. They grow by means of glandular secretion and epithelial desquamation. Complications include rupture of the cyst contents and rarely transformation to squamous cell carcinoma. Rupture can cause chemical meningitis, with potential sequelae of vasospasm, infarction and death.

These lesions are well defined, lobulated and of variable size. There is a thick capsule, which may contain calcification. The contents of the cyst are thick, foul-smelling, yellow material, possibly with hair and/or teeth. The liquid cholesterol gives the same signaling characteristics as fat (hyperintensity on T1, non-enhancement and heterogeneous appearances on T2). The appearances of a ruptured cyst are of fat droplets in the subarachnoid cisterns, sulci and ventricles. There may be associated pial enhancement from chemical meningitis.

Similar appearances may be seen with epidermoid, craniopharyngioma, teratoma and lipoma. Epidermoid cysts reflect the characteristics of cerebrospinal fluid and are usually found off the midline. Craniopharyngiomas are suprasellar, midline masses, but are hyperintense on T2 with strong enhancement. Teratomas are usually found in the pineal region. Lipomas show homogenous fat signal and also show a chemical shift artefact, which is not seen with dermoid cysts.

Reference

Osborn AG, Preece MT. Intracranial cysts: radiologic-pathologic correlation and imaging approach. *Radiology*. 2006; **239**(3): 650–64.

Case F

History

A 75-year-old male patient with shortness of breath

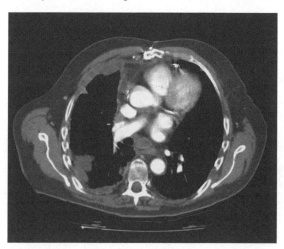

Figure i Arterial phase CT of the chest and abdomen (soft tissue window)

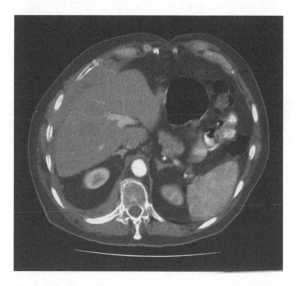

Figure ii Arterial phase CT of the chest and abdomen (soft tissue window)

Observations and interpretation

CT of the chest and abdomen (arterial phase):

- multiple enlarged mediastinal nodes, with necrotic subcarinal nodes and paracardiac nodes;
- circumferential nodular pleural thickening of the right hemithorax, extending onto the right pericardial surface and below the diaphragm into the right upper quadrant and through the chest wall into the subcutaneous soft tissues;
- on lung windows, the left lung appears normal with no evidence of parenchymal deposits;
- the right lung contains nodular soft tissue along the oblique fissure with volume loss of the right hemithorax;
- the portal venous scan shows several low-density lesions in the anterior aspect of the left lobe of the liver, which are suspicious for metastatic deposits or direct transdiaphragmatic extension;
- no evidence of bone metastases;
- the pancreas, spleen, kidneys and adrenals have normal appearances;
- previous median sternotomy and coronary artery bypass graft.

Main diagnosis

In view of the nodular soft tissue involvement of the pleural and peritoneal surfaces, mesothelioma would be the main diagnosis.

Differential diagnoses

Other primary malignancies can metastasise to the pleura, including primary bronchogenic and breast carcinomas.

Further management

- Referral to the Respiratory MDT meeting for discussion of further management
- Offer ultrasound/image-guided biopsy

Discussion

Malignant pleural mesothelioma is a relatively uncommon malignancy that generally occurs in the context of prior asbestos exposure. Presenting symptoms include dyspnea, chest pain, cough and weight loss. As demonstrated by this case, the neoplasm can invade both visceral and parietal pleura. The overall prognosis is poor, with poor prognostic factors including intrathoracic lymph node metastases, distant metastatic disease and extensive pleural involvement. Palliation involves radiotherapy. Multimodality treatment with surgery and chemoradiotherapy has been found to improve survival.

CT is used for staging using the TNM system. Important points include the distinction between T3 (potentially resectable, such a solitary focus involving the chest wall, but not involvement of the pericardium) and T4 (non-resectable, such as diffuse tumour extension or multiple chest wall foci, transdiaphragmatic extension, involvement of the pericardium). MRI is sometimes used for improved detection of tumour extension. PET can assist in determining nodal involvement, assessing for occult metastases as well as guiding biopsy by detecting the more metabolically active areas of the pleural disease.

Key features to assist in making the diagnosis on CT include unilateral pleural effusion, nodular pleural thickening, interlobar fissure thickening, calcified pleural plaques in 20%, contraction of the involved hemithorax with features of volume loss (mediastinal shift, narrowed intercostal spaces, elevation of ipsilateral hemidiaphragm). Signs of locally aggressive behaviour include invasion of the chest wall (loss of extrapleural fat planes, invasion of intercostal muscles, displaced ribs, bone lysis), mediastinum and diaphragm. Extrathoracic spread may be also be demonstrated on CT, including direct hepatic invasion, retroperitoneal extension and retrocrural adenopathy.

A tissue histological diagnosis is required to be certain of the diagnosis, as it can be difficult to distinguish malignant mesothelioma from metastatic adenocarcinoma or severe atypia on cytology alone. Thoracotomy or thoracoscopy guided biopsy can also help yield a tissue sample.

Mesothelioma can occur within the peritoneum alone in approximately 30% of cases. The association with asbestos is less in this subgroup than in those patients with pleural mesothelioma. CT appearances include ascites, peritoneal thickening and scalloping on adjacent abdominal organs. Other disease processes to consider in the context of diffuse peritoneal disease include papillary serous carcinoma of the peritoneum and desmoplastic small round cell tumour. Benign entities that occur include benign mesenchymal tumours (lymphatic, vascular, neuromuscular or fat in original tissue type). Malignant mesenchymal tumours can also occur, such as primary sarcomas of the subperitoneal space, the most common of which is the liposarcoma. Rarely, lymphoma and leukaemia can infiltrate the peritoneum – the former is known as peritoneal lymphomatosis.

References

Pickhardt PJ, Bhalla S. Primary neoplasms of peritoneal and sub-peritoneal origin: CT findings. *Radiographics*. 2005; **25**(4): 983–95.

Wang ZJ, Reddy GP, Gotway MB, *et al*. Malignant pleural mesothelioma: evaluation with CT, MR imaging, and PET. *Radiographics*. 2004; **24**(1): 105–19.

Paper 5

Case A
History
A 5-month-old with vomiting and colicky abdominal pain

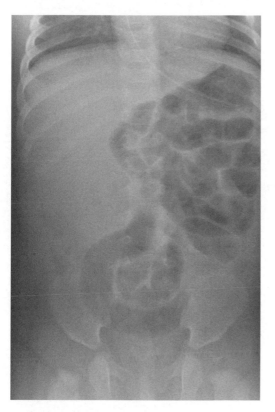

Figure i Abdominal radiograph

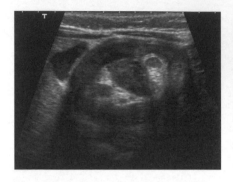 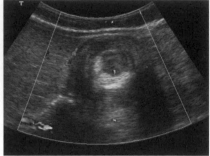

Figure ii Abdominal ultrasound, right upper quadrant transverse section

Figure iii Abdominal ultrasound, right upper quadrant transverse section

Observations and interpretation

Abdominal radiograph:
- small bowel obstruction;
- no gas in the large bowel;
- no pneumoperitoneum.

Abdominal ultrasound:
- right upper quadrant heterogeneous donut-shaped mass;
- lesion almost target-like;
- lymph nodes but no fluid noted within the lesion;
- Doppler flow demonstrated within the lesion;
- both kidneys appear normal, as do the rest of the solid organs;
- no free fluid.

Main diagnosis
Intussusception

Differential diagnoses
Mass related to bowel

Further management
- This is a surgical emergency – immediately inform the paediatric surgeons.
- May consider performing an abdominal radiograph to ensure a complication such as perforation has not already occurred and assess degree of obstruction.
- Once the child has been appropriately resuscitated, and usually with antibiotic cover, an attempt at hydrostatic or pneumatic reduction can be made.

Discussion
Intussusception is defined as the telescoping of one segment of the gastrointestinal tract into an adjacent one. It is relatively common in children and is the second most common cause of an acute abdomen and is the leading cause of acquired bowel obstruction in childhood. The peak incidence is between 6 months and 2 years of age. It is much less common in adults and accounts for less than 5% of cases of mechanical small bowel obstruction. Whereas the diagnosis is usually already suspected in children before imaging as they commonly present with a classic history of vomiting and red currant jelly stool, it is often made unexpectedly in adults. In addition, although in children there is usually no specific underlying cause, an underlying lead point is often present in adults.

In children the aetiology is usually idiopathic, probably secondary to mucosal oedema and lymphoid hyperplasia following a viral illness. Occasionally, intussusception can be secondary to a lead point – for example, a Meckel's diverticulum – but this is rare. The most common site is ileocolic followed by ileoileocolic, ileoileal and finally colocolic. It is a surgical emergency, as there is the potential for vascular compromise of the intussuscepted segment, which may lead to infarct and eventually perforation.

Plain film radiography, barium studies and ultrasound imaging play major roles in both the diagnosis and management of this condition in children. In experienced hands, ultrasound has both high sensitivity and specificity in the detection of intussusception. Classic findings on transverse scanning include a so-called 'target lesion' or 'crescent in doughnut sign', often with the presence of several concentric rings. The inner hypoechoic ring is formed by the intussusceptum, with the outer ring representing the intussuscipiens and an intermediate hyperechoic area indicating the space between. On longitudinal imaging, multiple thin parallel stripes of varying degrees of echogenicity with a sandwich-like appearance are typically seen, the so-called 'pseudokidney sign'. If peritoneal fluid is trapped inside the intussusception then this has an association with irreducibility and ischaemia. Colour Doppler can demonstrate the mesenteric vessels dragged into the lesion. Lack of Doppler flow is a concerning feature that suggests bowel necrosis. Patients demonstrating this may go for surgical intervention rather than attempted reduction.

On plain film there may be evidence of obstruction, a soft tissue mass or even a cresenteric sign – where a crescent of luminal gas outlines the apex of the intussusceptum. Antegrade contrast studies classically give a 'coiled spring' appearance. CT is rarely used in the paediatric population for assessment due to the radiation.

Attempted reduction uses either hydrostatic or pneumatic pressure, usually no greater then 120 mmHg. The success rate of reduction is operator dependent but in many departments is up to 90%. The exact methods and protocols used vary between institutions and according to the individual case but the rule of 3s is a common guide seen in many textbooks. Whether using hydrostatic or pneumatic reduction the rule of 3s is useful; maximum three attempts for 3 minutes each. The main contraindication to attempting reduction is perforation or strong evidence of bowel infarction, peritonitis or hypovolaemic shock. Unfortunately, there is a recurrence rate of up to 10%, complications rarely occur but include perforation, reduction of non-viable bowel and incomplete reduction.

Reference

Byrne AT, Geoghegan T, Govender P, *et al.* The imaging of intussusception. *Clin Radiol.* 2005; **60**(1): 39–46.

Case B

History

A 66-year-old male with worsening liver function test results and abdominal pain

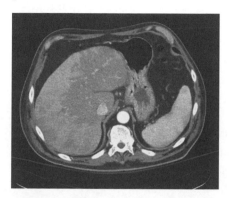

Figure i Arterial CT of the abdomen and pelvis

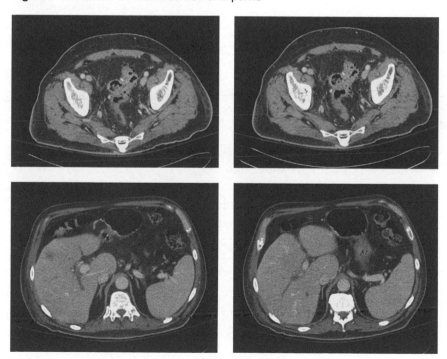

Figures ii–v Portal venous phase CT of the abdomen and pelvis

Observations and interpretation

CT of the abdomen and pelvis (arterial and portal venous phase):

- diverticulitis of the sigmoid colon accompanied by significant local inflammatory change;
- adjacent to the mid portion of the sigmoid is a small gas-containing collection, which is consistent with a localised perforation and abscess;
- thrombus in the right portal vein extending from the bifurcation;
- peripherally in the right lobe of the liver there are subtle areas of parenchymal low density, which is in keeping with oedema, but as yet there are no intrahepatic abscesses;
- no intrahepatic duct dilatation;
- the appearances of the rest of the solid organs are unremarkable bar renal cysts; the biliary tree is unremarkable;
- no further gastrointestinal abnormalities;
- the lung bases are clear bar atelectasis;
- no significant bony lesions.

Main diagnosis

Acute right portal vein thrombosis secondary to complicated diverticulitis

Differential diagnoses

Perforated sigmoid tumour with secondary portal vein thrombosis

Further management

- Urgent referral to appropriate surgical team
- Discussion with interventional radiologists regarding drainage of the pelvic abscess
- Team to discuss starting anticoagulation and antibiotics
- Radiological follow-up of the liver, particularly to ensure hepatic abscesses do not form in the areas of oedema – ultrasound may be the most useful modality for this in the first instance

Discussion

Diverticulosis is an extremely common condition, affecting the majority of people later in life. Diverticula can occur anywhere throughout the colon but are most common in the sigmoid. They represent small outpouchings of the colonic mucosa and submucosa through the muscular layers of the wall. The outpouchings occur mainly where the vessels pierce the muscularis, between the mesenteric and antimesenteric teniae. This relationship of the diverticula to the penetrating blood vessels explains the propensity of diverticula to bleed. At CT, diverticulosis appears as small air- or faeces-filled outpouchings of the colonic wall. The wall of the involved colonic segment may appear thickened because of muscular hypertrophy. These diverticula are predisposed to inflammation and thereby diverticulitis. Acute diverticulitis occurs when the neck of a diverticulum is occluded by stool, inflammation or food particles, resulting in a microperforation of the diverticulum and surrounding pericolic inflammation.

At CT, diverticulitis appears as segmental wall thickening and hyperaemia with inflammatory changes in the pericolic fat. The key to distinguishing diverticulitis from other inflammatory conditions that affect the colon (e.g. inflammatory bowel disease, ischaemia) is the presence of diverticula in the involved segment. Also, diverticulitis typically occurs in the descending or sigmoid colon. CT also allows detection of other complications of diverticulitis such as diverticular abscess, fistula formation (most commonly colovesical) and perforation. An abscess can be seen in up to a third of cases and appears as a fluid collection with surrounding inflammatory changes. When an abscess is detected, CT can also provide guidance for percutaneous drainage. Focal contained perforations can also be a complication of diverticulitis and appear as small extraluminal pockets of air or extravasation of oral contrast material. Generalised pneumoperitoneum is not a common finding in patients with diverticulitis. One potential pitfall of diagnosis of diverticulitis with CT is overlapping imaging findings in diverticulitis and colon cancer. In some cases it may not be possible to distinguish diverticulitis from colon cancer with CT alone, and histologic samples will be required to exclude an underlying malignancy.

Portal vein thrombosis occurs in various clinical settings, with the most common being liver cirrhosis. Other processes that may cause portal venous system thrombosis are inflammatory processes (e.g. diverticulitis, cholangitis, pancreatitis), neoplasms, hypercoagulable states, myeloproliferative disorders, surgery and embolism from a thrombus located in the superior mesenteric or splenic vein.

Colour Doppler ultrasound is the single most useful tool for detection of portal vein thrombosis. It is also useful for distinguishing between bland and neoplastic thrombosis. Unenhanced CT may show focal high attenuation in the portal, superior mesenteric, or splenic vein and venous enlargement when thrombosis is acute. Chronic venous thrombosis can manifest as linear areas of calcification within the thrombus. Contrast-enhanced CT demonstrates a filling defect partially or totally occluding the vessel lumen. Rim enhancement of the vessel wall may also be seen and is presumed to be due to normal flow in the vasa vasorum. Indirect signs of portal vein thrombosis are the presence of cavernous transformation of the portal vein and the presence of portosystemic collateral vessels and arterioportal shunts – the former are more associated with chronic thrombosis, as these larger collateral vessels take time to form. Care must be taken to avoid confusion of the 'pseudothrombus image' with a true portal vein thrombus. The pseudothrombus appearance occurs during arterial phase imaging and is due to mixing of unenhanced and enhanced venous flow. However, a homogeneously enhanced portal vein is seen during the portal venous phase.

Two types of perfusion anomalies have been reported in portal vein thrombosis: first, an arterialisation of the affected segments as arterial flow takes over the compromised portal venous flow; second, diminished enhancement during the portal venous phase. Portal vein thrombosis is usually treated by addressing the underlying cause if possible and by anticoagulation.

References

Gallego C, Velasco M, Marcuello P, *et al.* Congenital and acquired anomalies of the portal venous system. *Radiographics.* 2002; **22**(1): 141–59.

Horton KM, Corl FM, Fishman EK. CT evaluation of the colon: inflammatory disease. *Radiographics.* 2000; **20**(2): 399–418.

Case C

History

A 45-year-old female with left iliac fossa pain and history of left ovarian cyst

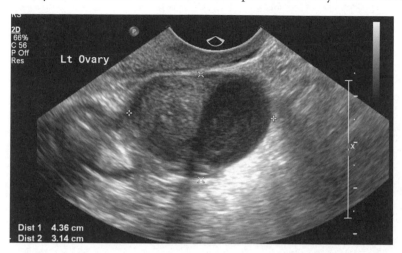

Figure i Transabdominal ultrasound of the left adnexa transverse section

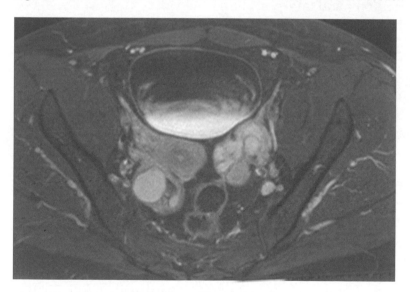

Figure ii Axial T1 fat-suppressed MRI

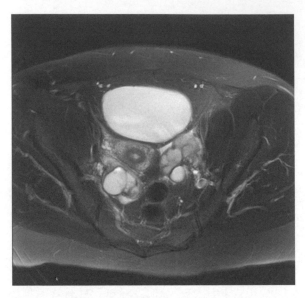

Figure iii Axial T2 BLADE fat-suppressed MRI

Observations and interpretation

Transabdominal and transvaginal ultrasound of the pelvis:

- the left ovary is large in volume and is expanded by the presence of multiple complex cysts, some of which have a mixed echogenic appearance;
- small amount of free fluid around the left ovary;
- the right ovary is more normal in volume but contains another small cyst;
- the uterus is anteverted with a poorly defined endometrium of 5 mm.

MRI of the pelvis:

- multiple bilateral adnexal cysts;
- most of these are high signal on T2- and T1-weighted sequences suggestive of haemorrhage breakdown products;
- several of the haemorrhagic cysts have thick walls;
- a few simple ovarian cysts are noted bilaterally;
- bilaterally the fallopian tubes appear distended with similar material seen in the cysts;
- mucus retention cysts are noted near the internal cervical os;
- no lymphadenopathy, only a trace of free fluid within the pelvis;
- bone marrow signal is within normal limits; incidental perineural cyst at L5/S1.

Main diagnosis

Endometriosis involving both adnexae, including the fallopian tubes and probably a plaque of endometroid tissue along the anterior rectum

Differential diagnoses

- Haemorrhagic ovarian cysts – this would not explain the involvement of the fallopian tubes
- Atypical tumour (e.g. desmoid tumour or some other mesenchymal tumour) – tumour can have a multitude of appearances

Further management

- Referral to Gynaecology and discussion at the relevant MDT meeting
- Tumour markers including CA-125

Discussion

Endometriosis is defined as encysted functional endometrial epithelium and stroma in an ectopic site outside the uterine cavity. This functional ectopic epithelium then undergoes the changes of the menstrual cycle causing local haemorrhage and inflammation. Common sequelae of endometriosis are called endometriomas; these are cysts that contain haemorrhagic break-down products from many menstrual cycles and are also sometimes known as 'chocolate cysts'.

Endometriosis is fairly common and occurs in 5%–10% of menstruating women and up to 5% of women on hormone replacement therapy. It usually manifests during the reproductive years, often causing chronic pelvic pain and infertility. Although findings at physical examination may be suggestive, imaging is necessary for definitive diagnosis, patient counselling and treatment planning. Transvaginal ultrasound and MRI are the imaging techniques that are most useful for preoperative disease mapping. Initial transvaginal ultrasound is a reliable technique for detecting and character-ising pelvic disease. MRI is indicated as a complementary examination in complex cases of endometriosis or where the diagnosis is in doubt. CT is not considered the primary imaging modality for evaluation of endometriomas because findings are non-specific.

Cysts with low-level internal echoes and echogenic peripheral foci on ultrasound are suggestive of endometriomas. Endometriomas may occa-sionally be multilocular with thin or thick septations as well as nodularity of the wall, and other cystic masses cannot be excluded.

MRI has high specificity for identifying endometriomas, which are char-acterised by high signal intensity on T1-weighted images and low signal intensity on T2-weighted images. This is a phenomenon that is referred to as 'shading' and results from cyclic bleeding, although haemorrhagic breakdown products can have variable signal characteristics. Extraovarian sites of disease include the serosal surface of the uterus, urinary bladder, ureters and fallopian tubes. Involvement of the intestinal tract is not uncommon and has diverse clinical manifestations. Occasionally, endometriosis may result in obstruction of the appendix, resulting in acute appendicitis. It can also implant in scars.

References

Bennett GL, Slywotzky CM, Giovanniello G. Gynecologic causes of acute pelvic pain: spectrum of CT findings. *Radiographics*. 2002; **22**(4): 785–801.

Chamié LP, Blasbalg R, Pereira RM, *et al*. Findings of pelvic endometriosis at transvaginal US, MR imaging, and laparoscopy. *Radiographics*. 2011; **31**(4): E77–100.

Case D

History
A 40-year-old female who fell onto outstretched hand

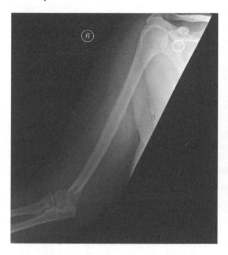

Figure i radiograph of the humerus

Figure ii CT of the humerus
(bone windows)

Observations and interpretation
Radiograph of the right humerus:
- at the level of the mid-diaphysis, there is a well-defined round area of calcification;
- the adjacent bone is normal in appearance, with no evidence of medullary lesion;
- no evidence of aggressive periosteal reaction (Codman's triangle or sunray spiculation);
- the lesion is solitary.

CT of the humerus (unenhanced):
- confirms that the area of ossification is within the adjacent soft tissues but not invading the overlying muscles (fat plane is visible);
- underlying bone is normal;
- the lesion is solitary;
- no evidence of an associated soft tissue mass or periosteal reaction.

Main diagnosis

In view of the non-aggressive features, myositis ossificans would be the primary diagnosis.

Differential diagnoses

None

Further management

- Review old films to assess for a previous injury
- Refer to Orthopaedics if symptomatic

Discussion

Extraskeletal osseous and cartilaginous lesions generally have quite characteristic radiological appearances and can therefore usually be distinguished. However, there is a spectrum of pathologies from which a differential diagnosis can be formed.

From the extraskeletal osseous tumours, myositis ossificans is the most common. It is a benign, solitary, self-limiting, ossifying soft tissue mass that is usually found within skeletal muscle and is of unknown pathogenesis. It can either occur in the setting of trauma or be non-traumatic (such as in paraplegics). The presentation can be either as an incidental finding or with pain and a soft-tissue mass. It is typically found in adults and most commonly in the large muscles of the extremities. There is no evidence that myositis ossificans is a premalignant condition, and local excision is curative in symptomatic patients.

There is a chronological pattern to both the histopathology and radiographic appearances of this process. Within 2–3 weeks of the onset of symptoms, faint calcification will be seen. By 6–8 weeks, a sharply circumscribed bony mass is usually present, which may decrease in size and mature by 5–6 months. Deep lesions may be associated with the periosteum but are usually separate from it with an intervening radiolucent zone. The key distinguishing feature (from more aggressive entities) is that of peripheral mature ossification.

The CT appearances demonstrate a rim of mineralisation around lesions after 4–6 weeks, with low attenuation centres. Diffuse ossification may be seen in more mature lesions. The MRI appearances also progress in a chronological pattern. In the early stages, the appearances are of a heterogeneous signal lesion, which is of increased signal relative to fat on T2-weighted sequences, with surrounding oedema. T1-weighted images show a lesion, which is isointense to skeletal muscle and relatively poorly defined. There may be curvilinear low signal peripherally, due to mineralisation. Intermediate lesions may have a more clearly defined peripheral low-signal rim of mineralisation. Fluid-fluid levels may occasionally be seen secondary to haemorrhage, although this is a non-specific feature and is seen with several other processes. Mature lesions are well defined and have signal intensities similar to fat, with surrounding low signal. As the lesions are vascular initially, enhancement is seen with intravenous contrast.

Bone scintigraphy has been used in the past to monitor the activity, with intense focal tracer uptake on both dynamic and blood pool imaging. Early on, the delayed images show mild uptake only, which subsequently increases and later decreases as the lesion matures.

There are a number of relatively uncommon variants, including myositis ossificans progressiva, panniculitis ossificans, fibro-osseous pseudotumour of the digits. A rare osteosarcoma, which occurs in the extraskeletal tissues, can have similar appearances to myositis ossificans. It generally occurs in an older age group (mean age, 50 years) and commonly with a history of prior irradiation. The presentation is usually of a painful, enlarging soft tissue mass, with cloud-like mineralisation seen on plain radiographs. There is no peripheral ossification as is seen with myositis ossificans.

Reference

Kransdorf MJ, Meis JM. From the archives of the AFIP: extraskeletal osseous and cartilaginous tumors of the extremities. *Radiographics*. 1993; **13**(4): 853–84.

Case E

History

A 20-year-old female with back pain

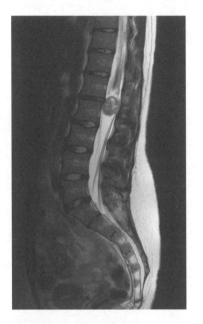

Figure i Sagittal T2 MRI

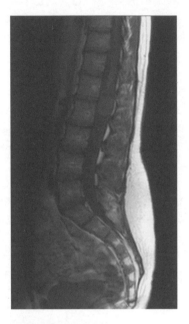

Figure ii Sagittal T1 MRI

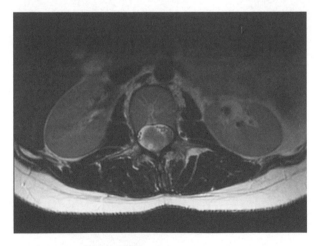

Figure iii Axial T2 MRI

Observations and interpretation

MRI of the lumbar spine (T1 and T2 sagittal, T2 axial):

- ovoid lesion seen within the spinal canal at the level of the L1/2 intervertebral disc;
- the lesion lies inferior to the conus and does not expand it, displacing it to the left of the spinal canal, together with the nerve roots of the cauda equine;
- the lesion lies within the spinal canal and is therefore intradural but extramedullary;
- the signal characteristics of the lesion are heterogeneous on T2 sequences and intermediate on T1;
- minor disc bulges at the lower four lumbar levels but no annular tears;
- loss of height of the L1/2 disc;
- cord signal is normal.

Main diagnosis

The lesion is intradural and extramedullary; therefore, metastases and neurofibroma would be possible.

Differential diagnoses

Unless there was a pre-existing central nervous system malignancy, metastases would be very unlikely in this age group.

Further management

- Recall for post-contrast imaging
- Recommend referral to a dedicated Spinal or Neurosurgical unit for MDT meeting discussion and further management

Discussion

This case was found to be a schwannoma and although screening for neurofibromatosis type 1 was performed, there was no conclusive evidence of this.

Within the spine, it is useful to categorise lesions into the following groups: (a) extradural, (b) intradural and extramedullary, and (c) intramedullary. Extradural lesions include prolapsed or sequestered disc, metastases, myeloma, lymphoma deposits, neurofibroma, meningioma, haematoma or abscess. Intradural lesions include meningioma, neurofibroma, metastases and subdural empyema. Intramedullary lesions include ependymoma, astrocytoma, dermoid, infarct and haematoma.

This is an extensive topic and warrants review in a general radiology textbook. However, in the intradural/extramedullary category, the most common differentials include meningioma, nerve sheath tumours and drop metastases. Meningioma is commonly found in the thoracic region, in women more than men. Neurofibromatosis should be thought of when multiple meningiomas are seen. CT and MRI characteristics are similar to those of intracranial meningiomas, with dense calcification sometimes seen, and dural tails. Schwannoma is the main differential; these often extend out through a neural foramen and lack a broad dural base.

Nerve sheath tumours, or schwannomas, are the most common intraspinal mass and usually occur sporadically. In the cervical and thoracic region, extension into the neural foramen is often seen, with both intra- and extraspinal components. In the lumbar region, schwannomas tend to remain within the dural sac. Schwannomas can undergo cystic degeneration and necrosis. Neurofibromatosis type 2 is associated with multiple meningiomas and schwannomas. Neurofibromatosis type 1 is associated with multiple neurofibromas, which can have a plexiform appearance in the spine.

Intrathecal or drop metastases can also be intradural and extramedullary in location. The typical cause for these is subarachnoid seeding of primary central nervous system tumours, including posterior fossa medulloblastomas, ependymomas and pineal region neoplasms. Other solid tumours, including breast and lung primaries can also metastasise to the subarachnoid space. MRI with gadolinium enhancement is used for screening the lumbar spine pre-operatively in these cases.

Reference

Gaensler, EHL. Nondegenerative diseases of the spine. In: Brant WE, Helms CA. *Fundamentals of Diagnostic Radiology*. 3rd ed. Philadelphia, USA: Lippincott Williams & Wilkins; 2007. pp. 271–321.

Case F

History

A 58-year-old male with strange feeling in skin

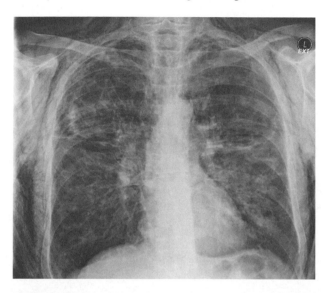

Figure i Chest radiograph

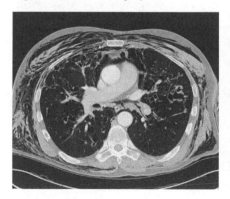

Figure ii Arterial phase CT of the chest (lung windows)

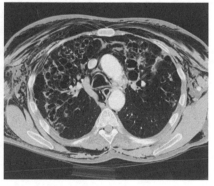

Figure iii Arterial phase CT of the chest (lung windows)

Observations and interpretation

Chest radiograph:
- right-sided pneumothorax with evidence of widespread surgical emphysema;
- the heart size is within normal limits;
- the right heart border is clearly defined, raising the possibility of a pneumomediastinum.

CT of the chest (arterial phase):
- widespread surgical emphysema and pneumomediastinum;
- subpleural bullae at both apices;
- thick-walled cysts at both bases, suggestive of an underlying abnormality such as cystic fibrosis;
- evidence of tree-in-bud at the left lower lobe, from possible infection;
- no evidence of an oesophageal injury.

Main diagnosis

Rupture of apical bulla with possible underlying cystic fibrosis

Differential diagnoses

Chronic obstructive pulmonary disease, although the cystic lesions would be atypical

Further management

- Referral to Chest physicians
- Discussion at the Lung MDT meeting regarding further management

Discussion

The causes of pneumomediastinum can be subdivided into intrathoracic or extrathoracic. Intrathoracic causes include a narrowed or obstructed airway, straining against a closed glottis, blunt chest trauma and alveolar rupture. Extrathoracic causes include sinus fracture, iatrogenic and perforation of a hollow visus (either peritoneal or retroperitoneal). The mediastinum is defined as the area between the thoracic inlet and the diaphragm. However, the mediastinum communicates with a number of anatomical structures, including the submandibular space, retropharyngeal space and vascular sheaths of the neck. There is also a communication to the retroperitoneum through the sternocostal attachment of the diaphragm, which extends to the flanks and pelvis. There is also a direct communication with the retroperitoneum via the periaortic and perioesophageal fascial planes.

The most common source of pneumomediastinum is from the terminal airspaces of the lung. Because of the pressure gradient, air from a ruptured alveolus passes into the perivascular and peribronchial fascial sheath. At the lung root, the fascial sheath also ruptures before a pneumomediastinum develops.

There are a number of radiographic signs of pneumomediastinum, including subcutaneous emphysema, thymic tail sign, pneumoprecardium (seen on a lateral chest radiograph), ring around the pulmonary artery, double bronchial wall sign, continuous diaphragm sign, extrapleural air and air in the pulmonary ligament. Particularly at the left heart border, it can be difficult to distinguish a medial pneumothorax from pneumo-mediastinum. In addition, normal overlying structures, such as fissure or the anterior junction line can simulate a pneumomediastinum. Chest CT is useful in confirming the presence or absence of pnemomediastinum or pneumopericardium. In addition, if there is no apparent underlying cause identified, CT may assist with identifying any lung parenchymal abnormali-ties or extrathoracic abnormalities.

Reference

Zylak CM, Standen JR, Barnes GR, *et al.* Pneumomediastinum revisited. *Radiographics*. 2000; **20**(4): 1043–57.

Paper 6

Case A

History

A 7-year-old male with acute and persistent swelling over right mandible

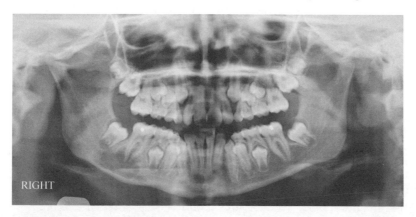

Figure i Orthopantomogram

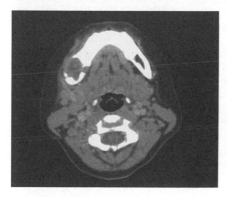

Figure ii Arterial phase CT
(soft tissue windows)

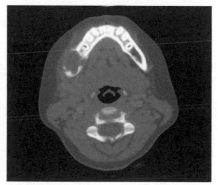

Figure iii Arterial phase CT (bone
windows)

Observations and interpretation

Orthopantomogram:
- well-defined lucent lesion in the right horizontal ramus of the mandible at the base of the right second molar causing a 'floating tooth' effect;
- this does not appear to breach the cortex;
- the lesion has a narrow zone of transition – no periosteal reaction is evident;
- this is a solitary lesion;
- no evidence of an associated soft tissue mass.

CT skull base and neck with contrast:
- expansile and lytic mass within the horizontal ramus of the right mandible and involving the roots of the second molar;
- expansion and destruction of the buckle cortex and a soft tissue component bulges through this to be limited by the buccinators, with a smaller defect in the lingual cortex;
- the zone of transition is narrow but there is a local periosteal reaction around the margins of the lesion extending some distance along the horizontal and ascending rami;
- overall these features are most in keeping with a lesion on the benign end of the spectrum;
- no lymphadenopathy;
- no lung lesions.

Main diagnosis

Eosinophilic granuloma – the features could be suggestive of a neoplasm, but the narrow zone of transition and lack of bony infiltration indicate that this may be a relatively benign process. This combination of atypical features supports the diagnosis of eosinophilic granuloma.

Differential diagnoses

- Primary bone neoplasm: these have a spectrum of appearances and can only be confirmed on biopsy.
- Infection/abscess formation: this should be clinically apparent and a less well-defined zone of transition might be expected.
- Fibrous dysplasia: although the presence of a periosteal reaction would be against this and the typical ground glass appearance is not present.
- Metastasis: unlikely in this age group and a more aggressive appearing lesion would be expected.
- Dentigenous cysts/cysts that occur in the jaw: unlikely, as the soft

tissue element, destructive nature and periosteal reaction would not be features of these benign cystic processes.

Further management

- Referral to Head and Neck surgeons, for discussion at MDT meeting and consideration of biopsy.
- MRI may be useful to further characterise the soft tissue component.

Discussion

Eosinophilic granuloma is one of the three main subtypes of Langerhans cell histiocytosis, a condition of unknown aetiology that is characterised by the proliferation of reticulohistiocytic elements. Eosinophilic granuloma accounts for up to 80% of Langerhans cell histiocytosis. It is a benign disease limited to bone or lung, with the majority having solitary lesions. It is most common in the age group of 4–8 years and it usually presents with pain and local swelling.

In the bones, eosinophilic granuloma can have a myriad of appearances which can sometimes make diagnosis challenging and it is often a diagnosis of exclusion. Most frequently it presents as a well-defined lucency in the medulla with or without endosteal scalloping or periosteal reaction. Punched out lesions can be seen in the skull and destructive lesions in the skull base, sellar, mastoids or mandible are also suggestive of this diagnosis. Lesions in the mastoid and mandible can lead to the characteristic appearance of 'floating teeth'. It is also the most common cause of solitary vertebrae plana in this age group.

A variety of management plans have been reported for solitary eosinophilic granuloma of bone, including observation, injections of steroid, local excision and curettage with or without bone grafting, chemotherapy and irradiation. All of these treatments are reported to give satisfactory results with a recurrence rate of less than 20%.

Reference

Hermans R, De Foer B, Smet MH, *et al.* Eosinophilic granuloma of the head and neck: CT and MRI features in three cases. *Pediatr Radiol.* 1994; 24(1). 33–6.

Case B

History

A 72-year-old with a history of weight loss, abdominal pain and night sweats

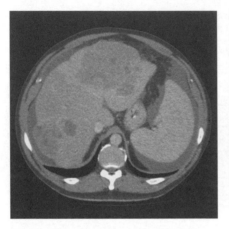

Figure i Portal venous phase CT

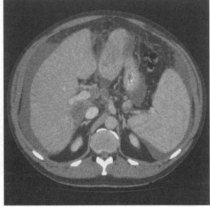

Figure ii Portal venous phase CT

Observations and interpretation

Portal venous phase CT of the abdomen and pelvis:

- hepatosplenomegaly;
- multiple ill-defined low-attenuation masses throughout the liver; the liver also has a slightly irregular surface;
- moderate- to large-volume ascites;
- no varices present, normal opacification of the portal vein;
- para-aortic and aortocaval lymphadenopathy;
- unremarkable gastrointestinal tract;
- appearances of the rest of the solid organs within normal limits (incidental prostate calcification);
- lung bases are clear;
- no significant bony lesions.

Main diagnosis
Lymphoma with extranodal involvement of the liver – this diagnosis is best fit with the presenting symptoms and the radiological appearances

Differential diagnoses
- Solid organ and lymph node metastases from an unidentified primary tumour – this would not explain the splenomegaly.
- Hepatic cirrhosis with associated hepatocellular carcinoma and portal hypertension causing splenomegaly – the liver is usually smaller in cirrhosis and there is no other evidence of portal hypertension.

Further management
- Refer to the appropriate Oncological or Haematological MDT meeting
- Complete the staging with a CT of the neck and chest, suggest tumour markers are obtained
- Consider ultrasound or MRI to characterise the hepatic lesions further
- Consider tapping ascites for biochemical and cytology analysis
- Discuss obtaining tissue for diagnosis, if no convenient nodal disease is identified on further imaging then biopsy of the liver lesions could be considered

Discussion
Lymphoma is usually divided into Hodgkin's and non-Hodgkin's disease. Hodgkin's lymphoma is responsible for approximately one-third of all lymphoma and is characterised histologically by the presence of Reed-Sternberg cells. Non-Hodgkin's lymphoma is a heterogeneous group of disorders with numerous subtypes and disease profiles. Lymphomas are also routinely categorised according to grade, ranging from slowly progressing, indolent disease to aggressive, fast-growing lesions.

Lymphoma most commonly affects the nodes and the spleen, causing lymphadenopathy and splenomegaly; occasionally, splenic involvement can manifest as focal lesions. Lymphoma frequently affects the liver but primary lymphoma of the liver is rare, secondary lymphoma is much more common, occurring in up 60% of patients with Hodgkin's and 50% in non-Hodgkin's lymphoma. There are several patterns of liver involvement; the most common is infiltrative, which can be difficult to detect on conventional imaging, and less frequently, a focal nodular pattern occurs. This is easier to detect on cross-sectional imaging. Rarely, a mixed pattern can occur.

STAGING OF LYMPHOMA

Stage I: Involvement of a single lymph node area

Stage II: Involvement of two or more lymph node areas on the same side of the diaphragm

Stage III: Involvement of lymph node regions on both sides of the diaphragm, with or without splenic involvement

Stage IV: Disseminated extralymphatic disease

CATEGORIES

Category A: B symptoms absent

Category B: B symptoms present

E: denotes extranodal disease with or without lymph node involvement.

CT is the mainstay for staging lymphoma and assessing response to treatment but functional imaging such as PET-CT is playing an increasingly important role in identifying occult disease and assessing metabolic as well as morphological response to treatment.

Reference

Fishman EK, Kuhlman JE, Jones RJ. CT of lymphoma: spectrum of disease. *Radiographics*. 1991; **11**(4): 647–69.

Case C

History

A 68-year-old female with symptoms of abdominal fullness and a pelvic mass on examination

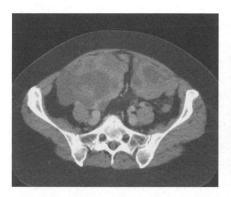 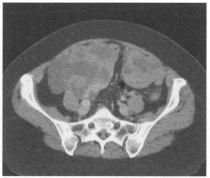

Figures i and ii Portal venous phase CT

Observations and interpretation

Portal venous phase CT of the abdomen and pelvis:

- bilateral large complex adnexal masses consisting of cystic and enhancing solid elements measuring approximately 20 × 13 cm; these appearances are highly suspicious of malignancy;
- small amount of free fluid in the pouch of Douglas;
- peritoneal nodule in left flank;
- 7 mm focal low-attenuation lesion within segment 5/8 of the liver – too small to characterise;
- the biliary system, pancreas, spleen, kidneys and adrenal glands are unremarkable;
- no lymphadenopathy;
- the lungs bases are clear;
- no significant bony abnormalities.

Main diagnosis

Bilateral ovarian cancer with extra-ovarian disease, probable stage III

Differential diagnoses

- Krukenberg's tumour from an unknown primary
- Appearances highly unlikely to be benign because of amount of abnormal enhancing soft tissue and the presence of peritoneal disease

Further management

- Urgent referral to the Gynaecology MDT meeting
- Suggest tumour markers are performed, including CA-125
- Discuss obtaining tissue; biopsy of the pelvic/peritoneal disease could be done under ultrasound or CT guidance
- Consider investigating other sites of primary disease if thought to be a Krukenberg's tumour
- If clinically indicated, further imaging of the small liver lesion possibly required

Discussion

Ovarian cancer is the most lethal of the gynecologic malignancies. Ovarian cancer symptoms are usually subtle and non-specific – therefore, the diagnosis is often delayed until the disease is well advanced. Overall 5-year survival is a rather dismal 50%, but this can be improved to greater than 90% if the disease is confined to the ovary at the time of diagnosis. Unfortunately, effective screening tools are currently not available. Incidence increases with age, with 80% of women diagnosed being over 50 years of age.

There are several histological subtypes. The most common are malignant epithelial tumours, which account for up to 85% of cases. Within this, there are further subcategories including serous, mucinous, endometroid and clear cell types. Other tumour types include malignant germ cell tumours and sex cord stromal tumours.

CA-125 can be useful in the work-up of these patients, as levels are elevated in up to 80% of patients with ovarian cancer; however, caution needs to be applied, as it can be positive in approximately one-third of benign disease processes.

Ultrasound is often used for initial assessment of patients with suspected disease and can be useful in characterising any focal lesions present. Suspicious appearances of masses on US include thick, irregular walls or septae, solid components, significant Doppler flow and large size. CT is the most routinely used modality to investigate and stage potential ovarian malignancy. CT can help characterise the primary lesion but also gives information on local extension, lymphadenopathy, involvement of local structures such as bowel, the presence of mesenteric, omental or peritoneal disease and other distant metastases. MRI is occasionally used to investigate and locally stage these patients – it combines the best features of both ultrasound and CT, giving superior tissue differentiation. Suspicious features on MRI are very similar to the other modalities; contrast is often used to identify abnormal enhancement, which can be very useful in the more subtle cases.

Despite the presence of imaging features that suggest malignancy, histopathology is usually required to rule out benign disease masquerading as malignancy and to guide treatment. Management of ovarian cancer depends not only on clinical and histopathological criteria but also, crucially, on stage. Staging is via TNM or FIGO classification.

FIGO CLASSIFICATION

Stage I
Growth limited to the ovaries

Stage IA
Growth limited to one ovary, no tumour on the external surface, capsule intact, no ascites present containing malignant cells

Stage IB
Growth limited to both ovaries, no tumour on the external surfaces, capsules intact, no ascites present containing malignant cells

Stage IC
Tumour either stage IA or IB, but with tumour on surface of one or both ovaries with capsule ruptured, with ascites present containing malignant cells, or with positive peritoneal washings

Stage II
Growth involving 1 or both ovaries with pelvic extension

Stage IIA
Extension and/or metastases to the uterus and/or tubes

Stage IIB
Extension to other pelvic tissues

Stage IIC
Tumour either stage IIA or IIB, but with tumour on surface of one or both ovaries, with capsule(s) ruptured, with ascites present containing malignant ovaries, or with positive peritoneal washings

Stage III
Tumour involving 1 or both ovaries with histologically confirmed peritoneal implants outside pelvis and/or positive retroperitoneal or inguinal nodes; superficial liver metastasis; tumour limited to true pelvis, but with histologically proven malignant extension to small bowel and omentum

Stage IIIA
Tumour grossly limited to the true pelvis, with negative nodes, but with histologically confirmed microscopic seeding of abdominal peritoneal surfaces or histologically proven extension to small bowel mesentery

Stage IIIB
Tumour of one or both ovaries with histologically confirmed implants, peritoneal metastasis of abdominal peritoneal surfaces ≤2 cm in diameter; nodes are negative

Stage IIIC
Peritoneal metastasis beyond the pelvis >2 cm in diameter and/or positive retroperitoneal or inguinal nodes

Stage IV
Growth involving 1 or both ovaries with distant metastases; if pleural effusion is present, positive cytology must be apparent to allot a case to stage IV; parenchymal liver metastasis qualifies as stage IV disease

Krukenberg's tumours are defined as secondary ovarian tumours from another primary – this is usually in the gastrointestinal tract. The most common is colon cancer, followed by stomach cancer. Two per cent of females with gastric cancer develop Krukenberg's tumours. These can have very similar appearances to primary ovarian malignancies and are bilateral in up to 85% of cases. This is another reason why biopsy of the lesion is important to give an accurate diagnosis and guide appropriate treatment.

Reference
Lutz AM, Willmann JK, Drescher CW, *et al*. Early diagnosis of ovarian carcinoma: is a solution in sight? *Radiology*. 2011; **259**(2): 329–45.

Case D

History
Thoracic back pain, previous colonic malignancy

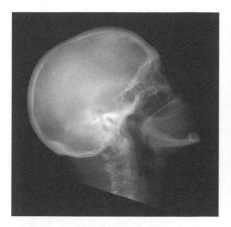

Figure i Skull radiograph

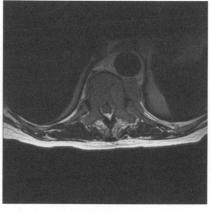

Figure ii Axial T2 MRI

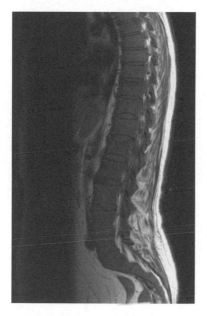

Figure iii Sagittal T1 MRI

Observations and interpretation

Skull radiograph:

- multiple round lytic lesions throughout the calvarium.

MRI of the thoracolumbar spine (T1/T2 sagittal and T2 axial sequences)

- soft tissue mass centred on lower thoracic spine, which is passing through a neural foreman on the right and displacing the spinal cord;
- further soft tissue mass anterior to the sacrum;
- diffuse low signal throughout the spine on T1-weighted images;
- superior endplate fracture at L1.

Main diagnosis

Multiple myeloma due to the punched-out lucencies and diffuse marrow involvement

Differential diagnoses

- Lytic bony metastases, although these would usually be more focal in terms of marrow involvement
- Haematological condition, such as myelofibrosis, lymphoma or leukaemia, in view of the widespread marrow involvement on MRI

Further management

- Referral to Haematology and discussion in the MDT meeting
- Urinary Bence-Jones proteins

Discussion

Multiple myeloma (MM) is a clonal B lymphocyte neoplasm of differentiated plasma cells. It is common and accounts for approximately 1% of all malignancies and about 10% of haematological malignancies. The median age at diagnosis is 65 years, with increased incidence in men and in African Americans. The aetiology of the disease is unknown, although there is an increased incidence post-irradiation.

Common presentations include fatigue, bone pain and symptoms relating to hypercalcemia. The key finding clinically is the detection in the blood or urine of the M protein, a monoclonal protein, which is produced by the abnormal plasma cells. Following positive results of these, a skeletal survey and bone marrow aspiration are performed, to assess for lytic lesions and plasma cells respectively. Seventy-five per cent of patients with MM will have positive radiographic findings, although it is estimated that approximately

50% of bone destruction must have occurred for it to be apparent on plain radiographs.

There are four forms of involvement by myeloma: (1) a solitary lesion (plasmacytoma), (2) diffuse skeletal involvement (myelomatosis), (3) diffuse skeletal osetopenia and (4) sclerosing myeloma. Plasmacytomas are lytic lesions that may be seen in the spine, skull, ribs, sternum and proximal extremities. Diffuse skeletal involvement is seen as osteolytic lesions, which are uniform in size and with distinct margins. Diffuse skeletal osteopaenia is typically seen at the spine and may result in compression fractures. Sclerotic lesions are less frequently seen and may be associated with POEMS syndrome (polyneuropathy, organomegaly, endocrinopathy, monoclonal gammopathy and skin changes).

MM on MRI is seen as hypointensities on T1-weighted images, hyperintensities on STIR, and enhancement after gadolinium administration, although these characteristics are not specific to MM. More indicative features include an expansile focal mass, multiple foci in the axial skeleton, diffuse marrow involvement or multiple compression fractures in a patient with no known primary malignancy. MRI is useful for monitoring post-treatment response.

Nuclear medicine bone scinitgraphy has a tendency to underestimate tumour burden because of the osteolytic (rather than osteosclerotic) nature of MM. However, PET-CT has recently been used for assessment of recurrence, as it can be used to image the whole body and it assesses functioning tumour tissue.

Reference

Angtuaco EJ, Fassas AB, Walker R, *et al.* Multiple myeloma: clinical review and diagnostic imaging. *Radiology.* 2004; **231**(1): 11–23.

Case E

History

A 46-year-old male, presented with sudden-onset right arm weakness

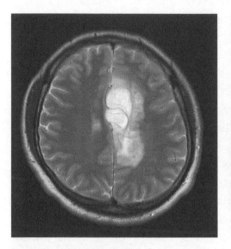

Figure i Axial T2 MRI

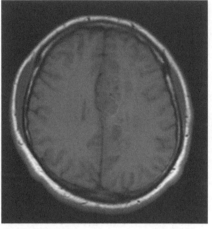

Figure ii Axial T1 MRI (pre-contrast)

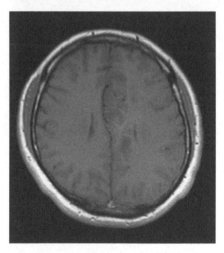

Figure iii Axial T1 MRI (post-contrast)

Observations and interpretation

MRI of the brain (T2 axial, T1 axial pre and post, T1 coronal):

- large lesion at the medial aspect of the left cerebral hemisphere, which extends to and crosses the midline;
- on T2 sequences, the lesion is mostly of intermediate signal with high signal cystic areas at the anterior aspect;
- the body of the corpus callosum is depressed and there is probable involvement by the lesion;
- minimal peripheral enhancement is demonstrated post contrast;
- no evidence of midline shift or hydrocephalus;
- the lesion is solitary.

Main diagnosis

A midline solitary lesion involving the corpus callosum, suggests a primary neoplasm is more likely, possibly an astrocytoma (which includes glioblastoma multiforme [GBM]) or primary lymphoma.

Differential diagnoses

- The location is very unusual for infection.
- Metastatic disease is unlikely because of the poor enhancement.

Further management

- A Neurosurgical and Neuro-oncological opinion is advised
- Referral to the Neuro-oncological MDT meeting
- Although less likely, review of previous imaging and medical history advised, to assess for an underlying primary malignancy

Discussion

There are a number of pathologies that affect the corpus callosum, including neoplastic (GBM, lymphoma, metastases), white matter disorders (multiple sclerosis, progressive multifocal leukoencephalopathy), acute shearing injuries, stroke and lipoma.

In adults, the most common supratentorial primary brain neoplasm is the astrocytoma, of which there are four subtypes: circumscribed (World Health Organization [WHO] grade I), diffuse (WHO grade II), anaplastic (WHO grade III) and GBM (WHO grade IV). The circumscribed types are more likely to occur in the posterior fossa. The diffuse types can occur anywhere in the brain, but quite commonly in the frontal and temporal lobes, with poor enhancement. They may demonstrate cystic change and calcification.

Anaplastic astrocytomas occur as transformed varieties of the lower-grade

119

lesions, and hence occur later in life. Features include poorly defined borders and extensive vasogenic oedema. They are more likely to enhance post contrast. Necrosis is a feature of a GBM rather than an anaplastic type. There is an approximately 50% transformation rate to GBM within 2 years.

GBMs can occur either *de novo* or from lower-grade astrocytomas. Overall, this grade is the most common subtype of astrocytoma, consisting of 50%–60% of all astrocytomas and 15% of intracranial tumours. The main feature on imaging is of necrosis. Higher grade is associated with increasing age, ring enhancement, enhancement of solid parts, marked mass effect and intratumoural necrosis. Typical features include crossing the corpus callosum, anterior or posterior commissure to invade the contralateral hemisphere. Because of the compact white matter tracts within the corpus callosum, oedema is rarely seen spreading across this structure. There may also be intratumoural haemorrhage and subarachnoid seeding.

One other type of astrocytoma to remember is the subependymal giant cell astrocytoma, which can occur in patients with tuberous sclerosis. These lesions are typically found near the foramen of Monro and have moderate or marked enhancement (unlike cortical tubers). They tend to project into the ventricular system and appear as a calcified mass. Other features associated with tuberous sclerosis include subependymal nodules and subcortical tubers.

Reference

Grossman RI, Yousem DM. *Neuroradiology: the requisites.* 2nd ed. Philadelphia, USA: Mosby; 2003.

Case F

History
A 58-year-old female with recurrent chest infections

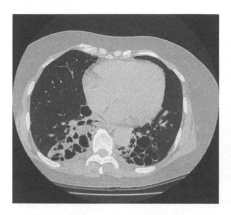 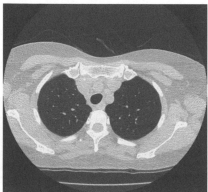

Figures i and ii Non-contrast CT (lung windows)

Observations and interpretation
Non-contrast CT of the chest with high-resolution CT supine images:
- no enlarged mediastinal or hilar nodes;
- the main pulmonary artery is enlarged in keeping with pulmonary hypertension;
- large cystic spaces within the posterior aspects of the lower lobes bilaterally and the lingular, in keeping with cystic bronchiectasis;
- no evidence of destructive bone lesions.

Main diagnosis
Cystic bronchiectasis with a background of small airways disease

Differential diagnoses
None

Further management
Referral to a respiratory physician for further management

Discussion
Bronchiectasis is defined as abnormal permanent dilatation of the airways, and can be subdivided into three types: (1) cyclindric, (2) varicose and (3) saccular (cystic). Cylindric is mild diffuse dilatation of the bronchi;

varicose is cystic bronchial dilatation with areas of narrowing, compared to a string of pearls; cystic bronchiectasis involves clusters of bronchi with localised saccular dilatation. Bronchiectasis can be defined as localised or generalised, with the localised type associated with previous infection, such as tuberculosis, and diffuse associated with an underlying condition such as cystic fibrosis. Conditions which predispose the bronchi to chronic inflammation can lead to bronchiectasis.

Plain radiographs of cystic bronchiectasis demonstrate multiple peripheral thin-walled cysts. Linear bronchial walls may be seen in other forms of bronchiectasis. On CT, cystic bronchiectasis can have an appearance like a bunch of grapes, a cluster of rounded lucencies, often containing air-fluid levels.

Cystic fibrosis is an inherited condition of young Caucasians, with the production of thick mucus, which leads to a cycle of recurrent infection. Haemoptysis can sometimes be a complication due to enlarged bronchial vessels. Bronchiectasis can also be found in dysmotile cilia syndrome, in particular Kartagener syndrome, the combination of sinusitis, situs inversus and bronchiectasis.

Severe childhood pneumonia with adenovirus, pertussis or measles can lead to bronchial damage, recurrent infection and ultimately bronchiectasis. Another pathogen that can cause bronchiectasis is the fungus *Aspergillus*. A hypersensitivity reaction to *Aspergillus* is known as allergic bronchopulmonary aspergillosis and is characterised by asthma, blood eosinophilia, bronchiectasis with mucus plugging and circulating antibodies to *Aspergillus* antigen. Patients usually have an underlying allergic history or cystic fibrosis. This tends to have an upper lobe predominance.

Reference

Klein JS. Airways disease. In: Brant WE, Helms CA. *Fundamentals of Diagnostic Radiology*. 3rd ed. Philadelphia, USA: Lippincott Wilkins & Williams; 2007. pp. 511–26.

Paper 7

Case A
History
A 2-year-old boy with a 3-month history of non-specific abdominal pain

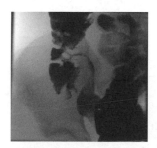

Figure i Fluoroscopic images of barium follow-through

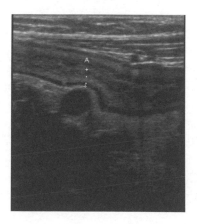

Figure ii US of the right iliac fossa

Observations and interpretation

Barium follow-through:

- the terminal ileum is narrowed and featureless, in keeping with a stricture;
- the ileum proximal to this narrowed segment is prominent which is consistent with pre-stenotic dilatation.

Abdominal ultrasound:

- thickening of the wall of the terminal ileum.

Main diagnosis

Terminal ileitis with structuring, most commonly due to Crohn's disease

Differential diagnoses

- Infective: this would be rare but can be indistinguishable from Crohn's – organisms include tuberculosis and *Yersinia*, among others.
- Inflammation: ulcerative colitis with backwash ileitis would be unlikely, as the colon appears normal.
- Neoplasia: occasionally lymphoma can mimic Crohn's ileitis, but this would be unusual in this age group.

Further management

- Referral to the Paediatricians
- Look for evidence of Crohn's complications (fistulae/sinuses)
- Consider MRI enteroclolysis/enterography to fully delineate the disease
- Consider repeat ultrasound after treatment to monitor response

Discussion

Crohn's disease is the most common inflammatory disease of the small bowel and most often involves the ileal or ileocaecal region; however, it can affect any part of the gastrointestinal tract.

The aetiology of this granulomatous inflammatory condition is currently poorly understood. The disease most often affects younger adults but it can affect the paediatric population and it also has a peak in later adulthood. It is a chronic condition with a wide variety of symptoms and potential complications. Paediatric Crohn's disease can be a serious and complex condition, which is not always easy to diagnose if it presents in an atypical manner. Although the pathological processes are the same in adults and children, the clinical presentation and disease distribution can be different in children.

The radiographic appearances are numerous but include aphthous ulceration (early sign), fissure ulcers, bowel wall thickening, 'cobblestoning', strictures and pseudosacculation. Features particularly indicative of Crohn's include aphthous ulceration, skip lesions and asymmetrical involvement. Complications often have high morbidity and include sinus/fistula formation, stricture and abscess formation. Longer-term complications include a significantly increased risk of gastrointestinal carcinoma or lymphoma. Associated conditions that are radiologically identifiable and are important to be aware of include enteropathic arthritis, sacroiliitis, cirrhosis/hepatitis, gallstones, renal calculi, cholangiocarcinoma and sclerosing cholangitis.

There are numerous radiographic techniques to investigate Crohn's – the most suitable depends on availability, indication and reducing radiation exposure, particularly important in the paediatric population. Commonly used techniques include contrast fluoroscopy, CT, MRI, ultrasound and capsule endoscopy.

Ultrasound can be very useful to identify and monitor bowel wall changes and to identify complications. MRI enterography is a clinically useful technique for the evaluation of both intraluminal and extraluminal small bowel disease. MRI enterography offers the advantages of multiplanar capability and lack of ionising radiation. It allows evaluation of bowel wall contrast enhancement, wall thickening, and oedema, findings useful for the assessment of Crohn's disease activity. However, endoscopic and fluoroscopic small bowel studies remain superior in the depiction of changes in early Crohn's disease.

References

Ali SI, Carty HM. Paediatric Crohn's disease: a radiological review. *Eur Radiol.* 2000; **10**(7): 1085–94.

Tolan DJ, Greenhalgh R, Zealley IA, *et al.* MR enterographic manifestations of small bowel Crohn disease. *Radiographics.* 2010; **30**(2): 367–84.

Case B

History

A 42-year-old male, readmission with right upper quadrant pain 10 days after an open cholecystectomy

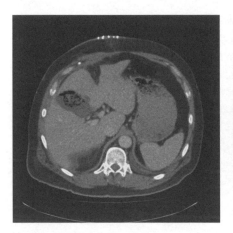
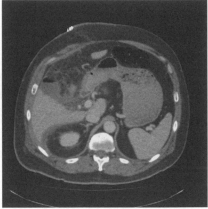

Figure i Portal venous phase CT   **Figure ii** Portal venous phase CT

Observations and interpretation

Portal venous phase CT of the abdomen and pelvis:

- contrast in large bowel from previous study;
- 7 × 3 cm fluid and gas collection in the gallbladder bed;
- fluid tracks around the top of the liver and to the retroperitoneum around the head of the pancreas;
- associated right upper quadrant inflammatory change;
- no free gas;
- other organs and gastrointestinal tract are essentially unremarkable;
- small, likely reactive, right pleural effusion with basal atelectasis.

Main diagnosis

Post-operative gallbladder bed collection

Differential diagnoses

- Bile duct injury/biloma – this cannot be totally excluded and should be suspected if the collection is drained and has bilious content.
- Duodenal/bowel injury – although the collection and inflammatory change are centred on the gallbladder fossa.
- Normal post-surgical appearances – this would be unlikely in an

uncomplicated operation as there is more fluid, gas and inflammatory change than would be expected for this interval post surgery. Equally, the clinical presentation suggests that this has not followed a normal post-operative course.

Further management

- Findings should be urgently reported to the referring team.
- Discussion with an interventional radiologist regarding insertion of ultrasound or CT-guided percutaneous drain.
- If clinically indicated, an MRI cholangiopancreatography or endoscopic retrograde cholangiopancreatography could be performed to investigate potential injury to the biliary tree.

Discussion

The main collection of fluid is seen in the gallbladder bed. This contains air – air would be not expected at this interval post-operatively and there is no air elsewhere in the abdomen. This strongly supports that the collection is infected and will likely require drainage.

Complication rates after cholecystectomy vary depending on a myriad of factors. These include whether the procedure was open or laparoscopic, whether it was performed acutely or electively, existing underlying inflammation and surgical experience.

The incidence of bile duct injuries is greater with laparoscopic procedures. These are serious injuries and early detection is crucial. Previously, the mainstay of investigation was scintigraphy, but now endoscopic retrograde cholangiopancreatography and MRI cholangiopancreatography are prevailing. Radiology also has a role in managing these injuries as biliary stent insertion is often preferably to surgical repair. Additionally, these patients require follow-up for many years to identify those who go on to develop strictures.

Reference

Connor S, Garden OJ. Bile duct injury in the era of laparoscopic cholecystectomy. *Br J Surg.* 2006; **93**(2): 158–68.

Case C

History

A 52-year-old male with a history of treated gastric carcinoid, now with ongoing weight loss

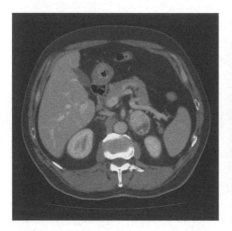

Figure i Portal venous phase CT   **Figure ii** Portal venous phase CT

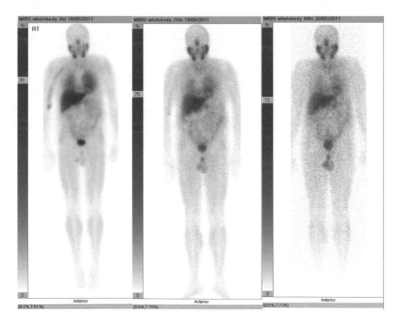

Figure iii MIBG study

Observations and interpretation

Portal venous phase CT of the chest, abdomen and pelvis:
- enhancing left adrenal mass measuring 4.5 cm;
- the right adrenal, liver, pancreas, spleen and kidneys are normal;
- no significant gastrointestinal tract appreciated, diverticulosis of the sigmoid colon;
- no lymphadenopathy;
- diffuse emphysematous lung changes but no suspicious pulmonary lesions;
- no suspicious bony lesions.

MIBG scan:
- intense tracer uptake in the left adrenal;
- no areas of extra adrenal uptake;
- the right adrenal is clear.

Main diagnosis

Phaeochromocytoma/adrenal paraganglioma

Differential diagnoses

- Neuroblastoma
- Metastasis from medullary cancer of the thyroid
- On the CT imaging alone, the differential is mainly between a phaeochromocytoma, a metastasis from carcinoid or another primary and lymphoma; the enhancement of the mass makes adenomatous change unlikely. The positive MIBG study precludes some of these diagnoses, leaving only those stated above in the main diagnosis.

Further management

- Referral to the relevant MDT meeting
- Measure urinary and plasma catecholamines
- Investigate clinically and perhaps radiologically whether the phaeochromocytoma is occurring as part of a syndrome

Discussion

The adrenal glands are composed of an outer cortex and an inner medulla that are functionally independent and distinct. The cortex secretes sex hormones and the medulla catecholamines.

Phaeochromocyotmas are rare tumours of the adrenal medulla that can occur at any age. They can cause symptoms of headache, hypertension and tremors due to overproduction of catecholamines, which can either be sustained or paroxysmal. Elevated urine vanillylmandelic acid is seen in approximately 50% of patients with a phaeochromocytoma. Occasionally phaeochromocytomas can present with significant haemorrhage, as they are the most common adrenal tumour to spontaneously bleed and the volume of haemorrhage can be very large.

Usefully, phaeochromocytomas generally follow the rule of 10:

- 10% are bilateral
- 10% are extra-renal
- 10% are malignant (these can metastasise to nodes, bone, liver and lungs)
- 10% are familial
- 10% are asymptomatic

Familial disease is associated with MEN IIa (medullary cancer of the thyroid, parathyroid adenoma and phaeochromocytomas) and IIb (medullary cancer of the thyroid, intestinal ganglioneuromatosis and phaeochromocytomas), von Hippel–Lindau's syndrome, neurofibromatosis I, tuberous sclerosis, familial phaeochromocytosis and Carney's syndrome.

Anatomical imaging of the adrenal glands is performed by ultrasound, CT and MRI. Most tumours are larger than 2 cm and can vary from cystic to solid. Calcification is rare but is classically eggshell when present. They show avid contrast enhancement and poor washout, which is a similar profile to adrenal metastases. Of note, non-ionic intravenous contrast can be used safety without alpha blockade.

Extra-adrenal sites of phaeochromocytomas include organ of Zuckerkandl, near the aortic bifurcation, and the para-aortic sympathetic chain. MRI can be useful in detecting atopic lesions as they usually demonstrate very high signal on T2-weighted images.

Functional imaging of adrenal disorders can be performed with I-131-MIBG scintigraphy. Cells of adrenal medullary origin such as phaeochromocytomas take up this isotope; MIBG in this instance is up to 90% sensitive and 99% specific. Additionally, neural crest tumours such as medullary thyroid cancer and neuroblastomas can concentrate MIBG. MIBG detects neuroblastomas and their metastases in over 90% of cases.

Treatment of phaeochromocytomas is via surgical removal under the cover of alpha and beta blockade. If the lesion has metastasised, then I131 MIBG can be used to target and treat metastases.

Reference

Van Gils AP, Falke TH, van Erkel AR, *et al.* MR imaging and MIBG scintigraphy of pheochromocytomas and extraadrenal functioning paragangliomas. *Radiographics.* 1991; **11**(1): 37–57.

Case D

History

Football injury 10 months ago, presents with 'locking' knee

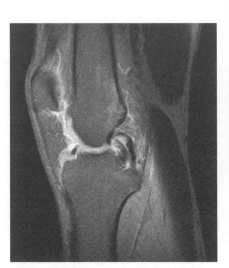

Figure i Saggital proton density fat-saturated MRI

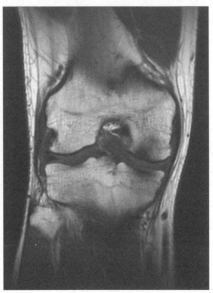

Figure ii Coronal T1 MRI

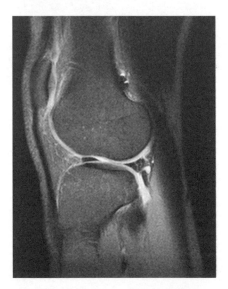

Figure iii Saggital proton density fat-saturated MRI

Observations and interpretation

MRI of the knee (proton density fat-saturated axial, sagittal and coronal sequences, T1 coronal sequences):

- joint effusion;
- complete tear of the anterior cruciate ligament (ACL);
- the posterior cruciate ligament (PCL) is intact;
- low-signal crescenteric fragment anterior to the PCL on the sagittal sequences, which is suspicious for a flipped meniscal fragment, consistent with a bucket handle tear of the medial meniscus;
- the lateral meniscus also has a complex tear of the posterior horn;
- low signal at the posterior medial femoral condyle is consistent with a bone contusion;
- no osteochondral fragments;
- cysts at the tibial spines, probably due to ACL avulsion;
- the medial collateral ligament is intact;
- the lateral collateral ligament and posterolateral structures are intact;
- the extensor mechanism is intact.

Main diagnosis

Full thickness ACL tear with flipped fragment of posterior horn medial meniscus in intercondylar notch.

Differential diagnoses

No differential diagnoses

Further management

Orthopaedic referral advised

Discussion

For imaging the acutely injured knee, plain films and MRI are the most useful investigations. MRI is useful in the context of rotational, valgus, varus or translation injuries. The pattern of abnormalities depends on the position of the joint at the time of injury. Imaging can be helpful when it is difficult to examine the knee clinically. A locked knee with restricted extension may be the result of muscle spasm associated with ligamentous injury (pseudolocking) or a true block from a displaced meniscus or osteochondral fragment. MRI can be used to distinguish these entities and direct the patient's management.

Plain film indications of significant soft tissue or bony injury include presence of a lipohaemarthrosis, lateral tibial casular avulsion fracture

(Segond lesion) or tibial spine avulsion fractures. MRI is required to assess the integrity of internal structures – in particular, assessment of patterns of injury.

In the context of a locked knee, the most common meniscal injury is a bucket handle tear, usually of the medial meniscus. This involves a large circumferential vertical tear with displacement of the free internal portion into the intercondylar region. On MRI, this is seen as a low-signal mass lying in the intercondylar notch, with the posterior part of the fragment lying under the PCL, producing the double PCL sign. The residual medial meniscus has an irregular edge and is smaller than normal. With a medial mensical injury, it is also important to assess the anterior cruciate ligament, and the medial collateral ligament for associated injuries.

Laterally, the posterior third of the meniscus can displace into the anterior compartment, which can look like an enlarged meniscus on several slices ('pseudohypertrophy'). It is important to assess for an attenuated posterior third in this context. A congenital discoid meniscus is a predisposing factor for tears of the lateral meniscus and this should be looked for, particularly in young patients.

Reference
Ostlere S. Imaging the knee. *Imaging.* 2003; **15**(4): 217–41.

Case E

History

An 85-year-old female with left-sided weakness

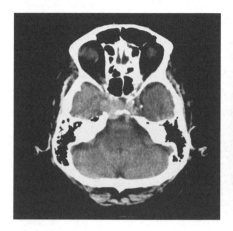

Figure i Pre-contrast CT

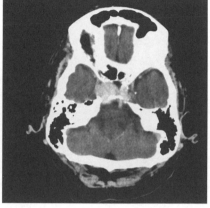

Figure ii Post-contrast CT

Observations and interpretation

Pre- and post-contrast CT of the head:
- at the medial aspect of the right middle cranial fossa, at the right cavernous sinus, there is a well-defined hyperdense area;
- this appears adjacent to the medial right temporal lobe, but not significantly compressing it;
- on the post-contrast scan, the lesion lies along the right internal carotid artery and is avidly enhancing;
- the right middle cerebral artery and other branches of the Circle of Willis are normal;
- there is minor involutional change consistent with the patient's age, with marked periventricular low attenuation, in keeping with small vessel disease;
- the optic nerves and sheaths are normal bilaterally;
- bone windows show slight expansion of the carotid canal just inferior to the lesion, but no hyperostosis or bone destruction;
- no evidence of intracranial blood, in particular subarachnoid blood.

Main diagnosis

A large aneurysm of the right internal carotid artery is the most likely diagnosis.

Differential diagnoses

A meningioma of the sphenoid wing could occur at this location, but a normal internal carotid artery would be expected separately.

Other pathologies at the cavernous sinus would include a trigeminal schwannoma or a vascular malformation.

Further management

- Discussion with Neurosurgeons as to further investigation and management
- Consider CT angiography or formal cerebral angiography

Discussion

Because of the range of structures located at the cavernous sinus, there are a number of pathologies that can occur here. These include vascular lesions, cavernous sinus meningioma, trigeminal nerve sheath tumour and other rare entities.

Vascular lesions include aneurysms, carotid-cavernous fistula and dural malformation. Aneurysms may erode the anterior clinoid processes and are associated with flow voids or mural thrombosis. MRI T1 sequences can be used to make the diagnosis and can be supplemented by MRA or catheter angiography. These aneurysms may cause mass effect on the cranial nerves within the cavernous sinus. Rupture of these aneurysms leads to creation of carotid-cavernous fistula (intradural aneurysms produce subarachnoid haemorrhage).

Carotid-cavernous fistula or dural malformations can enlarge the cavernous sinus, and may be associated with an enlarged superior ophthalmic vein. Thrombosis of the cavernous sinus can occur as part of a septic process or post procedure. Cavernous sinus meningiomas tend to follow the lateral margin of the cavernous sinus and may extend posteriorly along the tentorial margin. The signal characteristics are the same as meningiomas in other parts of the body.

Trigeminal schwannomas are rare and are predominantly based in the middle cranial fossa. On MRI, they are isointense on T1 and high signal on T2, with avid enhancement and regions of cystic change.

Reference

Grossman RI, Yousem DM. *Neuroradiology: the requisites*. 2nd ed. Philadelphia, USA: Mosby; 2003.

Case F

History

Chronic lung disease, smoker

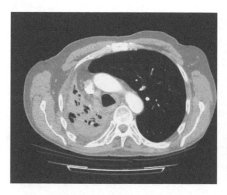

Figure i Arterial phase CT
(lung windows)

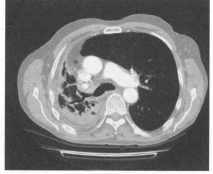

Figure ii Arterial phase CT
(lung windows)

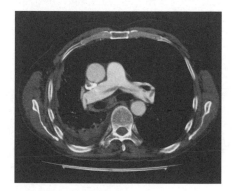

Figure iii Arterial phase CT
(soft tissue windows)

Observations and interpretation

Arterial phase CT of the chest:

- the trachea is deviated to the right secondary to volume loss in the right upper lobe;
- there is mediastinal lymphadenopathy;
- within the right upper lobe, there is dense collapse and consolidation with bronchiectasis;
- no endobronchial lesion is seen;
- bronchiectasis is also seen of the lower lobe;
- there are multiple pneumatoceles in the left lung;
- no discrete cavities are seen in the right lung;
- non-occlusive saddle embolus is also noted with flattening of the intraventricular septum;
- no bone lesions.

Main diagnosis

Non-occlusive saddle embolus and unilateral bronchiectasis affecting the right lung, suggestive of allergic bronchopulmonary aspergillosis

Differential diagnoses

Other causes of bronchiectasis

Further management

- Referral to a Respiratory physician for anticoagulation
- Review of previous imaging and enquiry about previous history of asthma/lung disease

Discussion

Aspergillus fumigatus, the organism that causes aspergillosis, is a ubiquitous soil organism that occurs commonly in the sputum of normal people. The different appearances within the lungs caused by this fungus depend on the immune status of the host. A hypersensitivity response leads to allergic aspergillosis, in normal patients, sacrophytic (non-invasive, with associated aspergilloma) aspergillosis can occur, with mild immunosuppression, chronic necrotising aspergillosis may be seen, and in severe immunosuppression, invasive pulmonary aspergillosis may manifest. In a pre-existing cavity, such as from previous tuberculosis infection, a fungus ball or mycetoma may develop.

In allergic bronchopulmonary aspergillosis, although this condition may start in young asthmatics, it may not become apparent until several decades later. Radiographic features include transient, alveolar subsegmental infiltrates in the upper lobes most commonly, central varicose or cystic bronchiectasis with 'finger in glove' mucus plugs, lobar consolidation, cavitation, hyperinflation and fibrosis. Blood markers include an eosinophilia and elevated serum IgE. The differential for impaction of dilated airways included, endobronchial lesions, bronchial atresia and bronchiectasis from other causes.

Saprophyic aspergillosis does not invade tissues, and although most patients are asymptomatic, the most common presenting symptom is haemoptysis. The characteristic feature is the 'air crescent' sign on both plain radiographs and CT, which reflects the soft tissue mass within a cavity. The mass, containing fungal hyphae and debris, moves on changing patient position.

Chronic necrotising (also known as semi-invasive) aspergillosis may occur insidiously in patients with chronic comorbidities such as diabetes, malnutrition, prolonged steroid treatment or increasing age. Radiographically, appearances include unilateral or bilateral segmental areas of consolidation, which may be associated with pleural thickening, nodular areas or cavitation. Appearances may progress over years.

Invasive aspergillosis usually affects small- to medium-sized pulmonary arteries and occurs in severely immunocompromised patients. CT findings include nodules, surrounded by a halo of ground-glass attenuation ('halo sign') or pleural-based wedge-shaped areas of consolidation, which correspond to haemorrhagic infarcts.

In view of these varied appearances, it is important to be aware of the possibility of underlying aspergillosis to enable appropriate treatment.

Reference

Franquet T, Müller NL, Giménez A, *et al*. Spectrum of pulmonary aspergillosis: histologic, clinical, and radiologic findings. *Radiographics*. 2001; **21**(4): 825–37.

Paper 8

Case A
History
A 3-day-old neonate with a left flank mass

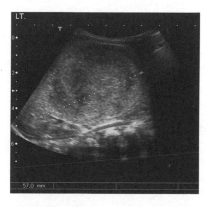

Figure i Abdominal ultrasound left upper quadrant

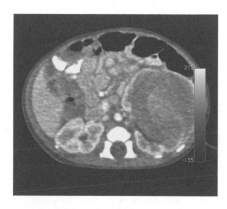

Figure ii Contrast-enhanced CT (soft tissue window)

Observations and interpretation

Abdominal ultrasound:

- large left-sided mass that appears to be arising from the left kidney, minimal normal parenchyma remaining;
- the remaining normal parenchyma appears around the mass in a 'claw like' shape;
- the mass is moderately vascular and heterogeneous in echotexture.

Contrast-enhanced CT of the abdomen and pelvis:

- large heterogeneously enhancing mass in the left kidney;
- arises from the renal parenchyma and appears to be confined within the kidney;
- the remaining normal parenchyma appears around the mass in a 'claw like' shape;
- no extension across the midline;
- no clot within the left renal vein or inferior vena cava;
- the right kidney enhances normally and there is no focal renal mass on this side; the right renal vein is identified and appears patent;
- no lymphadenopathy;
- the rest of the solid organs are unremarkable;
- no gross bowel abnormalities;
- no significant pulmonary or bony lesions seen.

Main diagnosis

Congenital mesoblastic nephroma

Differential diagnoses

- Wilms' tumour or nephroblastoma can have very similar appearances radiographically, but they are extremely rare in neonates and tend to present at age 2–3 years.
- Neuroblastoma – this is the most common abdominal malignancy in the newborn, but this tumour does not have features to support this, as it does not cross the midline, encase vessels or contain calcification.
- (Nephroblastomatosis would be highly unlikely, as the imaging characteristics are different. This is usually seen as multiple bilateral discrete homogenous nodules usually within the cortex that causes generalised enlargement of the kidney.)

Further management
- Referral to Paediatric surgeons and discussion at MDT meeting
- Consider image-guided biopsy of the lesion

Discussion
Congenital mesoblastic nephroma is the most common solid renal tumour in the newborn. Originally thought to represent congenital Wilms' tumour, mesoblastic nephroma has now been recognised as a distinct entity, often referred to as fetal renal hamartoma or leiomyomatous hamartoma. However, like Wilms' tumours, mesoblastic nephromas arise from the metanephric blastema and radiologically these tumours can be indistinguishable.

They are usually identified within the first 3 months of life, with 90% of cases discovered within the first year of life, with a slight male predominance.

The most common clinical presentation is a palpable abdominal mass, with haematuria a less frequent manifestation. Some cases are detected at prenatal ultrasound and may be associated with polyhydramnios, hydrops, premature delivery, and increased renin levels.

Radiographic features are of a solid, very large intra-renal mass in the neonate. This usually involves the renal sinus and replaces the majority of normal parenchyma. It may contain cystic, haemorrhagic or necrotic regions and local infiltration of peri-nephric tissue is common.

Although considered benign, mesoblastic nephromas can occasionally undergo sarcomatous transformation. These are usually successfully treated with nephrectomy alone but a wide surgical margin is necessary due to the infiltrative nature of the lesion. Rarely, the lesion may recur locally if incompletely resected or metastasize to the lungs, brain or bones. It is currently recommended that patients be closely followed up for 1 year after surgical resection. The prognosis is best if the tumour is diagnosed and resected before 6 months of age.

Reference
Lowe LH, Isuani BH, Heller RM, *et al.* Pediatric renal masses: Wilms tumor and beyond. *Radiographics.* 2000; **20**(6): 1585–603.

Case B

History

A 32-year-old female with acute abdominal peritonitis

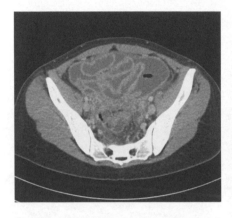

Figure i Portal venous phase CT

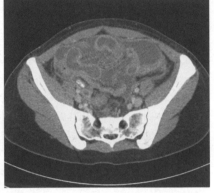

Figure ii Portal venous phase CT

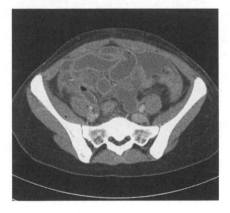

Figure iii Portal venous phase CT

Observations and interpretation

Portal venous phase CT abdomen and pelvis:

- large collection containing gas in the anterior lower abdomen;
- local peritoneal enhancement and wall thickening of adjacent small bowel loops;
- further collection is seen in the pouch of Douglas extending in a U shape around the uterus;
- extending into the pouch of Douglas collection is a dilated (up to 13 mm) fluid- and gas-filled appendix; this also contains an appendicolith and distal to this the wall is difficult to delineate, which is highly suspicious of perforation;
- inflammatory change is seen in the right iliac fossa and paracolic gutter;
- no further gastrointestinal tract abnormalities are appreciated;
- the solid organs appear within normal limits;
- the lung bases are clear;
- symmetrical sclerosis of the iliac portions of the sacroiliac joints, with minor sclerosis of the sacral component; although both joints appear normal and are not fused.

Main diagnosis

Appearances most consistent with perforated appendicitis with associated intra-abdominal collections.

Differential diagnoses

- There is no direct radiological evidence to support inflammatory bowel disease or caecal diverticulosis but these should always be considered when there is inflammation in the right iliac fossa. Additionally changes around the sacroiliac joints raise the possibility of background inflammatory bowel disease.
- There is no evidence that this is a secondary appendicitis – for example, due to an obstructing caecal tumour.

Further management

Urgent referral to the general surgeons

Discussion

Acute appendicitis is one of the most common causes of acute abdominal pain. Patients present with right lower quadrant pain, nausea and vomiting, and often have an elevated white cell count. CT has long been recognised as having a high diagnostic accuracy in patients with acute appendicitis with sensitivity and specificity of up to 95%. CT is usually performed in the portal venous phase with intravenous contrast. In addition, positive oral contrast may also be given, as this can elegantly demonstrate wall thickening but unfortunately may obscure an appendicolith, which would be a clue to the diagnosis.

A dilated, fluid-filled appendix is the most specific CT finding in acute appendicitis. Calcified appendicoliths and periappendiceal inflammation are helpful secondary findings. Enhancement of the appendiceal wall is often seen following intravenous contrast administration and is another specific sign of inflammation. Of note, in patients with adequate intraperitoneal fat, diagnosis can be made without oral or intravenous contrast material because the focal nature of the periappendiceal stranding is obvious.

CT can also demonstrate complications of appendicitis, including perforation, small bowel obstruction, and mesenteric venous thrombosis. Many other conditions can lead to inflammation and abscess formation in the right lower quadrant and mimic findings of acute appendicitis both clinically and radiologically – these include Crohn's disease and caecal diverticulitis. Essentially, all inflammatory processes of the gastrointestinal tract, including inflammatory bowel disease and infectious enteritis and colitis, can manifest with pain and produce inflammatory stranding in the mesenteric fat. One must be certain that the appendix is the cause of inflammation before making the diagnosis of acute appendicitis.

Based on current opinion, most patients with suspected or possible appendicitis should undergo cross-sectional imaging. CT scanning is preferred in most patients but US is recommended in children or pregnant women. MRI is usually indicated in women or children with non-diagnostic ultrasound.

Case C

History

A 74-year-old male with poor voiding

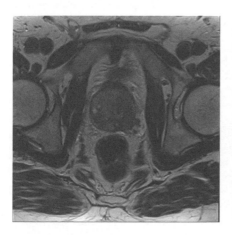

Figure i Axial T2 MRI

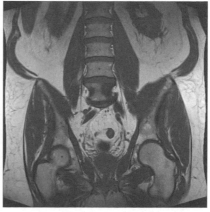

Figure ii Coronal T1 MRI

Observations and interpretation

MRI of the prostate (axial and coronal T2, coronal and sagittal T1, diffusion-weighted imaging):

- prostate is moderately enlarged due to transition zone benign prostatic hypertrophy;
- diffuse low signal in the prostate involving both peripheral zones and the left transition zone;
- the majority of this shows restricted diffusion;
- extracapsular tumour extension of low signal at the left prostatic base and bilateral seminal vesicle invasion;
- 18 mm in diameter soft tissue nodule within the bladder lumen is contiguous with the prostatic base and presumably represents a benign median lobe nodule;
- lymphadenopathy within the pelvis and para-aortic region of the abdomen;
- multiple areas of abnormal bone marrow signal in the posterior pelvis and vertebral column.

Main diagnosis

Diffuse bilateral prostate carcinoma with extracapsular tumour extension on the left side, bilateral seminal vesicle invasion, regional and non-regional lymph node disease and metastatic bone disease, which if confirmed on the subsequent biopsy would represent radiological stage T3b N1 M1b disease.

Differential diagnoses

This is extensive prostatic carcinoma until proven otherwise.

Further management

- Referral to Urological MDT meeting
- If biopsy not already performed then consider transrectal ultrasound biopsy
- Suggest performing serum prostate-specific antigen levels
- Consider performing a bone scan to further identify further bony metastases

Discussion

Prostate cancer is the most frequently diagnosed cancer in males and the second leading cause of cancer-related death in men. Adenocarcinoma is the most common histopathology; rare types include transitional cell cancer and adenoid cystic cancer.

Biopsy is important, as pathological grading determines treatment. This is done using the Gleason score (2–10) – this is the sum of the two most common histopathological patterns. A Gleason score ≥7 has a considerably worse prognosis than lower-graded tumours.

Assessment of prostate cancer can be divided into detection, localisation, and staging; accurate assessment is a prerequisite for optimal clinical management and therapy selection. MRI has been shown to be the gold standard in the local staging of prostate cancer. Traditional prostate MRI has been based on morphologic imaging with standard T1- and T2-weighted sequences, which has limited accuracy. Recent advances include additional functional and physiologic MRI techniques such as diffusion-weighted imaging, MRI spectroscopy and perfusion imaging. These techniques are useful as areas of tumour usually show restricted diffusion, have a particular biochemical composition and demonstrate increased vascularity. This provides information beyond anatomic assessment. Multiparametric MRI, combining these modalities, provides the highest accuracy in diagnosis and staging of prostate cancer. CT does not provide sufficient soft-tissue contrast within the prostate to evaluate local disease but CT can be valuable in the evaluation of pelvic lymphadenopathy and bone metastases. However, the combination of local MRI and bone scans have been found be most accurate for initial staging.

On MRI, the tumour is typically low signal on T2 and more intermediate on T1 sequences. Tumour is usually found in the peripheral zone of the gland but care should be taken to look for central tumours, although interpretation in this region is more difficult. The presence of benign prostatic hypertrophy also makes interpretation more challenging. In these circumstances diffusion-weighted imaging or dynamic contrast-enhanced MRI can be extremely useful and is now being more routinely performed.

Extracapsular extension can be difficult to delineate if there is small volume disease. Capsular thickening, focal bulging, flattening of the rectoprostatic angle, obliteration of fat planes, asymmetry of the neurovascular bundles are all indicators of extracapsular disease. The seminal vesicles are frequently involved. In younger patients the seminal vesicle are well hydrated and the presence of abnormal low signal can be easily appreciated; in older patients the vesicles can become dehydrated which can make detecting disease difficult; again this is where advanced MRI techniques can be very helpful. Local nodal staging is done by MRI, although this relies on the assessment of size and morphology that implicitly has limited sensitivities and specificities.

Reference

Bonekamp D, Jacobs MA, El-Khouli R, *et al.* Advancements in MR imaging of the prostate: from diagnosis to interventions. *Radiographics.* 2011; **31**(3): 677–703.

Case D

History
A 14-year-old with short stature

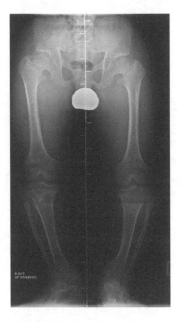

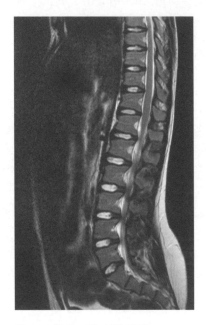

Figure i Whole-leg radiograph

Figure ii Sagittal T2 MRI

Observations and interpretation

Whole-leg radiographs:
- the long bones (femora, tibiae and fibulae) are short, with flared metaphyses;
- the iliac crests are squared and the acetabulae are shallow;
- the pelvic inlet has a 'champagne glass' configuration.

MRI of the lumbar spine (sagittal T1 and T2, axial T2):
- there are short pedicles and posterior scalloping of the vertebral bodies;
- the anteroposterior diameter of the spinal canal is reduced causing canal stenosis;
- normal bone marrow signal.

Main diagnosis
Achondroplasia

Differential diagnoses
None

Further management
Review of previous imaging and correlation with clinical findings

Discussion
Achondroplasia is an autosomal dominant, rhizomelic short-limbed dwarfism, most cases of which are due to spontaneous mutations. This form is one of the most common dwarfisms (1 in 26000 live births). Intelligence and life span are normal. Clinically, the patients demonstrate a protuberant forehead, lumbar kyphosis in infancy that progresses to an exaggerated lordosis in adults, and reduced elbow extension.

There are a number of distinguishing radiographic features. The skull is enlarged with narrowing of the foramen magnum. In the spine, there are bullet-shaped vertebrae in infancy, progressing to platyspondyly in adulthood, and narrowed interpedicular distance with short pedicles. The chest radiograph may show short ribs. In the pelvis, key features are squared iliac wings, horizontal acetabular roofs, and a narrow pelvic inlet, described as a 'champagne glass'. The long bones are short and wide, with flared metaphyses, In the hands, the appearance has been described as a 'trident', because of equal length of the second, third and fourth fingers. Neurological impingement, from spinal and cranial stenosis, is the main cause of morbidity.

Reference
Manaster BJ, May DA, Disler DG. Skeletal dysplasias. In: Manaster BJ, May DA, Disler DG. *Musculoskeletal Radiology: the requisites*. 3rd ed. Philadelphia, USA: Mosby; 2007. pp. 622–42.

Case E

History
55 year old female, headaches, vomiting

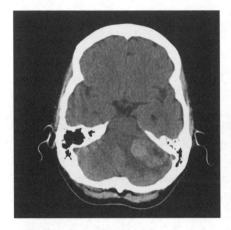

Figure i Pre-contrast CT

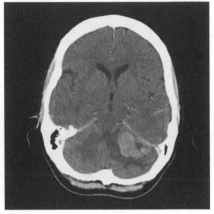

Figure ii Post-contrast CT

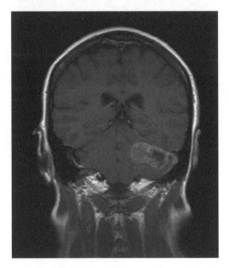

Figure iii Coronal post-contrast T1 MRI

Observations and interpretation
CT brain (pre and post contrast)
- There is a large soft tissue density mass at the left posterior fossa, which has central low density, due to necrosis, and enhancement of the soft tissue components post-contrast.

- It is difficult to be certain whether the lesion is intra or extra-axial.
- There is local mass effect with effacement of cerebellar folia, vasogenic oedema, displacement of the vermis to the right, partial effacement of the fourth ventricle and complete effacement of the quadrigeminal cisterns.
- The venous sinuses, in particular the left transverse sinus, enhance normally.
- No evidence of other lesions or lytic bone lesions.

MRI (pre and post contrast)
- The lesion at the left posterior fossa is noted, located posterior to the IAM (internal auditory meatus).
- It has a broad dural contact and is separate to the neural bundle at the IAM.
- The lesion is of heterogenous signal on T1 and T2 with high signal central areas on T2, representing fluid, and surrounding vasogenic oedema.
- There is distortion of the left middle cerebellar peduncle and partial effacement of the fourth ventricle.
- There is enhancement of the peripheral part of the mass and along the adjacent dura.
- No other lesions are seen.

Main diagnosis
In view of the age of the patient, even for the atypical location, a solitary metastasis is most likely.

Differential diagnoses
An acoustic neuroma can have similar appearances but the nerves at the left IAM have normal appearances.

A large meningioma (with necrotic centre) is a possibility.

Primary brain malignancies can occur in the posterior fossa but are less common in adults than children.

Further management
Urgent referral to Neurosurgery in view of raised intracranial pressure.

Review of past medical history for underlying primary malignancy.

Chest radiograph and breast examination/mammography, followed by staging CT chest, abdomen, pelvis if required.

Discussion

This patient was known to have had a previous breast malignancy and a recent staging CT also showed liver and lung metastases.

In adults, the most common infratentorial neoplasms are metastases. These tend to be well defined, round and typically located at the grey-white matter border. These lesions enhance post-contrast and may have nodular or ring enhancement. The most common primaries that metastasise to the posterior fossa are bronchial and breast, followed by melanoma, renal and thyroid. CT appearances are usually of low density lesions. MRI appearances are variable. However, haemosiderin may be identified in haemorrhagic lesions, including metastases from lung and breast, as well as primary neoplasms including, glioblastoma multiforme and oligodendroglioma.

With lung and breast brain metastases, it is also important to think about dural spread and subarachnoid seeding. Breast malignancy is the most common to be associated with purely dural disease. Adjacent bone lesions can also spread inwards to the dura.

The most common lesions at the cerebellopontine angle are vestibular schwannoma (previously called acoustic neuroma, and reflect the most common origin from the superior vestibular branch of cranial nerve VIII, 75%), meningioma (10%) and epidermoid (5%). There are a number of features to assess to distinguish between schwannoma and meningioma at this location. Meningiomas frequently exhibit a dural tail, have adjacent bony hyperostosis, calcify in 20% of cases, rarely exhibit necrosis, demonstrate uniform enhancement, rarely extend into the IAM, are hyperdense on nonenhanced CT and rarely bleed. Schwannomas rarely have a dural tail, calcification or elicit any bone reaction. They demonstrate necrosis in up to 10% of cases, make an acute angle with the dura and demonstrate heterogenous enhancement. On precontrast CT, they appear isodense and are more likely to haemorrhage. On MRI, schwannomas are usually iso- to hypointense relative to pontine tissue, with homogenous enhancement in 70% of cases.

Reference

Grossman RI and Yousem DM. *Neuroradiology: the requisites.* 2nd ed. Philadelphia, USA: Mosby; 2003.

Case F

History

Adult short of breath with lethargy, underlying chronic condition, and poor renal function

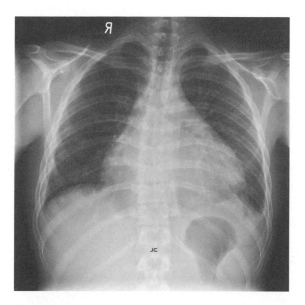

Figure i Chest radiograph

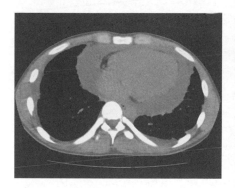

Figure ii Unenhanced CT (soft tissue windows)

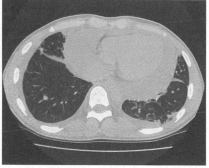

Figure iii Unenhanced CT (lung windows)

Observations and interpretation

Chest radiograph:
- the heart is enlarged and has a rounded contour, suggestive of a pericardial effusion;
- small bilateral pleural effusions;
- no focal lung lesions.

Non-contrast CT of the chest:
- large simple pericardial effusion and shallow bilateral pleural effusions;
- enlarged nodes in the superior mediastinum;
- the heart chambers are not dilated;
- ill-defined nodules seen at both bases, with surrounding ground-glass opacity.

Main diagnosis

Pericardial and pleural effusions with normal-sized heart are suggestive of a connective tissue disorder.

Differential diagnoses

The basal nodules could be due to infection or malignancy.

Further management

- Review previous imaging and clinical history for underlying cause
- If haemodynamically compromised, urgent referral to Cardiology for pericardiocentesis

Discussion

Pericardial effusions can be identified on plain radiographs and echocardiograms; however, CT and MRI are increasingly being used for identifying haemorrhagic pericardial effusions, constrictive pericarditis and pericardial masses. The pericardium comprises the parietal and visceral layers, which are separated by a small amount (15–50 mL) of serous fluid. The broad categories of conditions affecting the pericardium include infection, neoplasm, trauma, primary myocardial disease and congenital conditions. On cross-sectional imaging (CT and MRI), the normal pericardium should measure 2 mm or less, and it is best appreciated by the density differential with pericardial fat or fluid. The pericardial is generally seen over the right heart chambers, but not over the lateral and posterior walls of the left ventricle. There are several recesses, which can be identified as fluid density structures and may be misinterpreted as lymphadenopathy.

Pericardial effusions are typically thought to be due to obstruction of venous or lymphatic drainage from the heart, with underlying conditions including heart failure, renal insufficiency, infection, neoplasm (carcinoma of lung, breast, lymphoma) and injury (trauma or myocardial infarction). CT or MRI can be helpful for evaluation of loculated or haemorrhagic effusion, for assessment of pericardial thickening, or if further information is required following echocardiogram. On CT, it is useful to assess the density of any pericardial effusion. Fluid density of water is suggestive of a simple pleural effusion. If the effusion is of increased density, this could represent malignancy, haemopericardium (due to trauma or full thickness myocardial infarction), purulent exudate or effusion associated with hypothyroidism.

This patient was known to have systemic lupus erythematosus, a connective tissue disorder of autoimmune aetiology, which often affects the thorax. Thoracic disease may be limited to the pericardium and pleura and is due to a fibrinous serositis, which produces painful exudative effusions. The pleural effusions resolve with corticosteroid therapy. Pleural fibrosis and chronic thickening may occur in long standing disease. Pulmonary involvement may involve an acute lupus pneumonitis (which radiographically appears as rapidly coalescent bilateral airspace opacities) or chronic interstitial disease. Chronic fibrosis is relatively uncommon, however, and consideration of underlying mixed connective disease should be made.

Similarly, pulmonary involvement in the other connective tissue disorders (rheumatoid, scleroderma, dermatomyositis, polymyositis, Sjögren's syndrome and ankylosing spondylitis) occurs, most commonly with vasculitis and interstitial fibrosis.

References

Klein JS. Diffuse lung disease. In: Brant WE, Helms CA. *Fundamentals in Diagnostic Radiology*. 3rd ed. Philadelphia, USA: Lippincott, Williams & Wilkins; 2007. pp. 479–510.

Wang ZJ, Reddy GP, Gotway MB, *et al*. CT and MR imaging of pericardial disease. *Radiographics*. 2003; **23**: S167–80.

Paper 9

Case A

History

Infant with unexplained respiratory symptoms

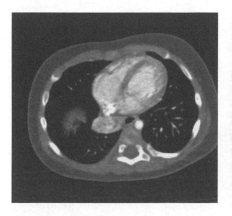 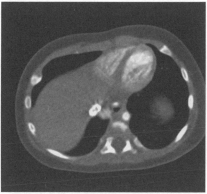

Figure i Arterial phase CT   **Figure ii** Arterial phase CT

Observations and interpretation

CT chest and upper abdomen arterial phase:

- 2 cm avidly enhancing soft tissue density within the right lower lobe abutting the diaphragm;
- this lesion has a systemic vascular supply arising from the coeliac axis and venous drainage to the pulmonary system;
- cystic regions of lung just posterolateral to the soft tissue lesion;
- aorta left-sided with a conventional branching pattern;
- two pulmonary arteries and four pulmonary veins are noted;
- appearances consistent with a congenital cystic lung abnormality.

Main diagnosis

Right lower lobe sequestration with arterial supply from the coeliac axis and pulmonary venous drainage (intralobar).

Differential diagnoses

Other congenital cystic lesions of the lung, congenital cystic adenomatoid malformations, bronchial atresia and bronchogenic cysts (these are unlikely, as this case has the classic characteristics of sequestration; however, in some cases these conditions can co-exist).

Further management

- Inform referring team/paediatric surgeons
- Investigate any potential associated congenital abnormalities

Discussion

Congenital lung anomalies vary widely in their clinical manifestation and imaging appearance. Although radiographs play a role in the incidental detection and initial imaging evaluation in patients with clinical suspicion of congenital lung anomalies, cross-sectional imaging such as CT is frequently required for confirmation of diagnosis, further characterisation and pre-operative evaluation in the case of surgical lesions.

Congenital cystic lesions of the lung comprise a heterogeneous group of bronchopulmonary malformations including congenital cystic adenomatoid malformations, sequestrations, bronchial atresia and bronchogenic cysts. Many lesions are now detected antenatally by prenatal ultrasound but they can also present in the postnatal period and, rarely, in later life. A pathology-based classification system has evolved; however, there remains controversy as to the degree of overlap between entities. It has been suggested that a common pathogenetic mechanism is responsible for the whole spectrum of lesions.

Pulmonary sequestration accounts for approximately 5% of all congenital pulmonary malformations so is therefore quite rare. This is defined as a segment of lung parenchyma that is separated from the tracheobronchial tree and is supplied with blood from a systemic rather than a pulmonary artery. It occurs predominantly in the posterobasal segments of the lower lobes, left more than right. The blood supply usually comes from the descending thoracic aorta, but in about 20% of cases it comes from the upper abdominal aorta, usually the coeliac artery or splenic artery. The pathway by which venous drainage takes place, however, varies depending on the type of pulmonary sequestration.

There are two types of pulmonary sequestration: extralobar sequestration (25%) and intralobar sequestration (75%). While extralobar sequestration is invested in its own pleura, intralobar sequestration manifests within the lung but without its own pleura. While there is general agreement that extralobar sequestration is congenital, there is some controversy regarding whether intralobar sequestration can be acquired via recurrent infections.

Over 50% of intralobar sequestrations may be asymptomatic by the time the patient reaches 20 years of age. In 95% of cases, venous drainage is to the pulmonary veins, resulting in a unique left-to-left shunt. Intralobar sequestrations are associated with other anomalies (usually diaphragmatic hernia) in about 15% of cases.

Extralobar sequestrations are contained within a distinct visceral pleural coat. This prevents collateral air drift, so the mass is usually airless in comparison with intralobar disease. Only 10% of extralobar sequestrations remain asymptomatic, and most present in the first 6 months of life. More than 80% drain into the right side of the heart via the azygos vein, hemiazygos vein, and inferior vena cava. They can even drain via the portal vein, left subclavian vein or the internal mammary vein. All these result in a left-to-right shunt. In 65% of extralobar sequestration cases there are associated anomalies, the most common being diaphragmatic hernia and congenital heart disease. Approximately a quarter of cases are associated with congenital diaphragmatic hernia and cystic adenomatoid malformation. Other pulmonary associations include lobar emphysema and bronchogenic cysts.

Rare variants of sequestration such as bilateral sequestration and gastric or oesophageal lung have been reported in both extra- and intralobar sequestrations. Where there is communication with the oesopahgus or stomach these are termed bronchopulmonary foregut malformations.

Imaging plays an integral part in the diagnosis and preoperative planning of sequestration. Appearances on chest radiograph include hyperinflation of the aerated lung, soft tissue masses, recurrent pneumonias and cavitatory or cystic lesions (intralobar only). The most common radiographic finding in patients with sequestration is a focal lung mass, almost always located in the lower lobes, with the left side more frequently involved than the right side. In symptomatic patients with intralobar sequestration, inflammatory changes due to recurrent infections are usually seen. Intralobar sequestrations that have been complicated by chronic inflammation and recurrent infection often evolve into predominately cystic lesions as air can drift into the affected segment due to the lack of intervening pleura. CT angiography with three-dimensional reconstruction is particularly helpful, not only for detecting anomalous arterial vessels, which aids in reaching an accurate diagnosis, but also in evaluating anomalous veins for differentiating between intralobar and extralobar sequestration. Most intralobar sequestrations require lobectomy or at least a segmentectomy of the involved lung. In contrast, an extralobar sequestration with its own lung pleura can be excised without resection of the normal lung.

References

Konen E, Raviv-Zilka L, Cohen RA, *et al*. Congenital pulmonary venolobar syndrome: spectrum of helical CT findings with emphasis on computerized reformatting. *Radiographics*. 2003; **23**(5): 1175–84.

Lee EY, Boiselle PM, Cleveland RH. Multidetector CT evaluation of congenital lung anomalies. *Radiology*. 2008; **247**(3): 632–48.

Case B

History

A 71-year-old female with microcytic anaemia, presumed gastrointestinal blood loss but normal oesophago-gastro-duodenoscopy and colonoscopy

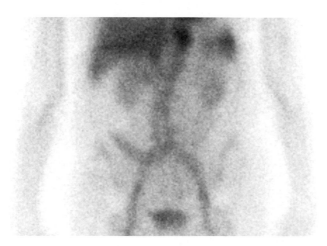

Figure i Nuclear medicine gastrointestinal bleed scan

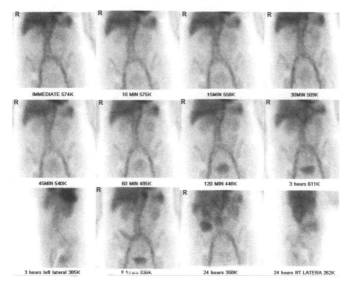

Figure ii Nuclear medicine gastrointestinal bleed scan

Observations and interpretation

Nuclear medicine gastrointestinal bleed scan:

- the important features are seen on the 6- and 24-hour images;
- activity is seen on the 6-hour film in a loop of bowel placed to the right of the midline, this would suggest activity is sited within distal small bowel;
- activity noted in the right colon on the 24-hour film;
- no abnormal activity seen elsewhere.

Main diagnosis

Ongoing small volume distal small bowel haemorrhage – this is can be secondary to numerous causes (*see* Discussion)

Differential diagnoses

Colonic haemorrhage

Further management

- Urgent report to referring clinician.
- If not already performed, consider CT mesenteric angiography or even interventional mesenteric angiography – the latter if there is haemodynamically significant haemorrhage, as embolisation may be required.
- If not already performed, consider standard staging CT abdomen and pelvis to look for underlying lesions or evidence of malignancy.
- Consider repeat colonoscopy and ileoscopy if the distal ileum was not well visualised previously; capsule endoscopy may also be useful.

Discussion

Gastrointestinal bleeding can be investigated in a number of ways – this depends on imaging availability and clinical factors but also crucially on the rate of bleeding itself. Endoscopy is usually the first line but this can often be negative in intermittent bleeding or if bleeding is within the small bowel.

Scintigraphy with technetium 99m-labelled red blood cells or technetium 99m-labelled sulphur colloid can be used to detect bleeding rates of more than 0.2 mL per minute. Sensitivity varies depending on rate of blood loss but is over 90% for blood loss greater than 500 mL per 24 hours; specificity is usually over 95%.

CT angiography is usually performed in triple phase with pre-contrast, arterial and delayed phases. Multidetector CT with its speed, resolution, multiplanar techniques and angiographic capabilities allows excellent visualisation of both the small and the large bowel. It can also demonstrate active bleeding into the bowel and is helpful in the acute setting for characterisation and visualisation of the bleeding source. Clot on pre-contrast imaging or extravascation of contrast into the lumen is diagnostic. This technique can detect bleeding rates of greater than 0.3 mL per minute.

Less favourable in the first instance, unless the patient is bleeding heavily enough to require intervention, is conventional angiography. This is obviously an invasive technique but it has the advantage of potentially treating as well as recognising gastrointestinal haemorrhage. This can identify bleeding rates of over 0.5 mL per minute.

The causes of small bowel bleeding are numerous and vary with patient parameters (e.g. age). Aetiologies include ulcers (benign or malignant), tumours (leiomyoma, adenomas and haemangiomas), vascular lesions (namely, telangiectasia and angiodysplasia), inflammation (including inflammatory bowel disease), varices, a Meckel's diverticulum, other diverticular, metastatic disease and amyloid pathology. Some of these processes could be recognisable on CT or MRI but many may require direct visualisation.

References

Geffroy Y, Rodallec MH, Boulay-Coletta I, *et al*. Multidetector CT angiography in acute gastrointestinal bleeding: why, when, and how. *Radiographics*. 2011; **31**(3): E35–46.

Holder LE. Radionuclide imaging in the evaluation of acute gastrointestinal bleeding. *Radiographics*. 2000; **20**(4): 1153–9.

Case C

History

A 62-year-old female with unexplained pelvic pain

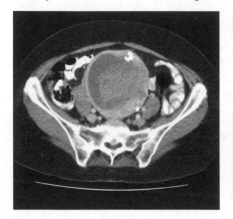
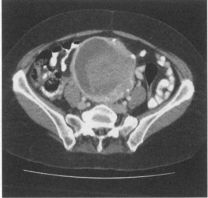

Figure i Portal venous phase CT   **Figure ii** Portal venous phase CT

Observations and interpretation

Portal venous phase CT of the abdomen and pelvis:

- the uterus is bulky with several calcified fibroids;
- irregular solid mass in the fundus that is suspicious for malignancy;
- fluid and a small bubble of gas in the endometrial cavity;
- the margins of the uterus remain well defined and the adjacent fat normal;
- the cervix appears unremarkable;
- no lymphadenopathy, ascites or peritoneal thickening/nodularity;
- the liver, pancreas, spleen and adrenal are unremarkable, as is the gastrointestinal tract;
- both kidneys have mildly full pelvicalyceal systems and ureters, apparently due to direct pressure on the distal ureters from the uterine mass;
- multiple nodules in the lungs, most conspicuous in the right lower lobe, which are highly suspicious of metastases;
- no suspicious bony lesions.

Main diagnosis
Endometrial carcinoma with probable pulmonary metastases (stage IVB)

Differential diagnoses
- Uterine sarcoma – this is much rarer than endometrial carcinoma
- Cystic degeneration/haemorhage into a fibroid uterus – this would not explain the pulmonary lesions

Further management
- Referral to the Gynaecological MDT meeting
- Consider further local staging with MRI
- Discuss obtaining biopsy, probably via hysteroscopsy
- Discuss potential interval imaging of the pulmonary lesions

Discussion
Endometrial carcinoma most commonly presents with abnormal uterine bleeding, usually postmenopausal, although it can present with other pelvic symptoms or symptoms related to metastatic disease. Most patients presenting with post-menopausal bleeding have a benign cause such as endometrial atrophy, endometrial polyps and non-uterine causes. Endometrial carcinoma accounts for up to 15% of cases of postmenopausal bleeding.

STAGING OF CARCINOMA OF THE ENDOMETRIUM

IA: Tumour confined to the uterus, no or <½ myometrial invasion
IB: Tumour confined to the uterus, >½ myometrial invasion
II: Cervical stromal invasion, but not beyond uterus
IIIA: Tumour invades serosa or adnexa
IIIB: Vaginal and/or parametrial involvement
IIIC1: Pelvic node involvement
IIIC2: Para-aortic involvement
IVA: Tumour invasion bladder and/or bowel mucosa
IVB: Distant metastases including abdominal metastases and/or inguinal lymph nodes

---

CT is a useful staging investigation in endometrial cancer, although it has obvious limitations relating to local staging. In this case CT was utilised not as a staging tool but for diagnostic purposes for unexplained symptoms.

Transvaginal ultrasound is a useful modality in evaluating patients with post-menopausal bleeding and other pelvic symptoms. Ultrasound signs of endometrial carcinoma include heterogeneity and irregular endometrial thickening. However, these signs are non-specific and ultrasound cannot reliably distinguish between benign proliferation, hyperplasia, polyps and cancer.

MRI gives excellent tissue differentiation and is extremely useful in characterising uterine pathology. The normal zonal uterine anatomy is clearly delineated on T2-weighted imaging. Endometrial carcinoma typically is isointense to myometrium on T1-weighted sequences and lower signal intensity than endometrial lining on T2-weighted sequences. Tumours are usually of lower signal intensity than the brightly enhancing normal myometrial tissue after contrast medium administration, and on dynamic contrast enhancement tumour enhances more slowly than the myometrium.

Fibroids, or leiomyomas, are the most common disorder of the uterus, having been reported in up to a quarter of women over the age of 30 years. Ultrasound findings are usually diagnostic, with sonohysterography and MRI imaging playing supplemental roles for further characterisation as needed. CT is not the primary modality for diagnosing or evaluating fibroids; however, fibroids are often found incidentally at CT – therefore, familiarity with their various CT appearances is important. Uterine enlargement with associated focal masses, which may be submucosal, intramural or subserosal in location, and uterine contour deformity are the most common CT findings. Hyaline degeneration is the most common secondary change seen in fibroids – degeneration may be so extensive that the leiomyoma appears predominantly cystic and may become quite large, thereby it can be confused with other uterine or ovarian disease. Solid 'mass-type' calcifications in a uterine mass are the most specific signs for leiomyoma. Subserosal and submucosal leiomyomas may become pedunculated and may undergo torsion of the pedicle with subsequent infarction, degeneration, necrosis and, potentially, infection. When a leiomyoma is submucosal in location, it can be easy to confuse with endometrial disease on CT; ultrasound or MRI may allow delineation of the distorted but otherwise normal endometrium.

Reference

Barwick TD, Rockall AG, Barton DP, *et al*. Imaging of endometrial adenocarcinoma. *Clin Radiol*. 2006; **61**(7): 545–55.

Case D

History

A 47-year-old female with a swollen right calf

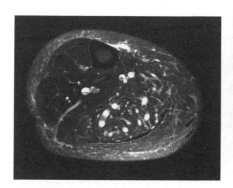

Figure i Axial T2 fat-saturated MRI

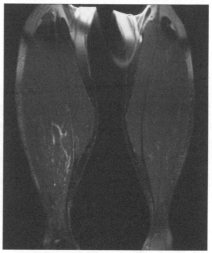

Figure ii Coronal T2 fat-saturated MRI

Observations and interpretation

MRI of both lower legs (T1 coronal, T2 fat-saturated sagittal, coronal and axial):

- within the right soleus muscle, there are multiple high T2 signal serpiginous areas, which are due to multiple dilated vessels;
- they arise from the posterior tibial and peroneal vessels;
- the muscle is enlarged but the signal is normal;
- the bone marrow signal of the tibia and fibula is normal;
- there is no soft tissue mass demonstrated.

Main diagnosis

In view of the multiple dilated vessels, the appearances would be most in keeping with a vascular malformation.

Differential diagnoses

None

Further management
Referral to a Vascular MDT meeting for discussion of further management

Discussion
Peripheral vascular (also known as arteriovenous) malformations can be difficult to diagnose and treat. Clinically, they can be asymptomatic or be a cause of high output cardiac failure. Surgery has classically been the method of management but this can have complications. Therefore, interventional techniques have been explored. There have been a number of classifications proposed, but a commonly used one relates to the grade of flow and the subsequent management. Therefore, slow flow lesions can be treated by sclerotherapy, intermediate flow by sclerotherapy with embolisation, and high flow by embolisation with sclerotherapy.

Vascular malformations are congenital lesions, which only manifest because of thrombosis, infection, trauma or endocrine changes. In contrast to haemangiomas, they grow in proportion with the patient. As haemangiomas involute over time, definitive treatment is usually not required. The pathology is of aberrant vessel angiogenesis, with direct connections between arteries, veins and lymphatic vessels, without a normal capillary bed. A nidus is the confluence of small tortuous vessels, where arteriovenous shunting occurs without a capillary bed. One vascular malformation can contain more than one nidus. A syndrome that involves multiple vascular malformations is Osler-Weber-Rendu syndrome.

Plain films can demonstrate bone and joint involvement. Phleboliths are seen in the context of haemangioma. Ultrasound can be used to assess arterial and venous velocities and monitor patients after treatment. CT is useful for assessing run-off, involvement of deep structures and concomitant lesions. However, MRI can provide the majority of this information without the radiation exposure. Slow flow malformations have high T2 signal on MRI, while high flow malformations have signal voids. Angiography is important prior to interventional procedures. Direct puncture of the nidus can provide information about the volume and flow pattern. A variety of agents are used for sclerotherapy, including ethanol, ethanolamine oleate and polidocanol. Following the procedure, follow-up should be clinical with imaging if required, to assess for recurrence.

Reference
Hyodoh H, Hori M, Akiba H, *et al.* Peripheral vascular malformations: imaging, treatment, approaches, and therapeutic issues. *Radiographics.* 2005; **25**(Suppl. 1): S159–71.

Case E

History

A 39-year-old female with an 18-month history of slowly enlarging mass

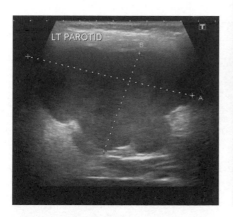

Figure i Ultrasound of the left parotid

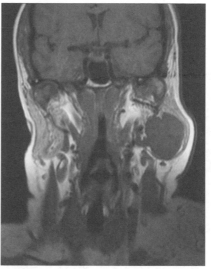

Figure ii Coronal T1 MRI

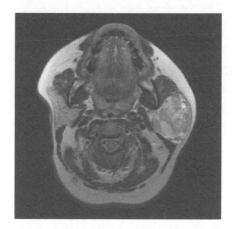

Figure iii Axial proton density MRI

Observations and interpretation
Ultrasound of the neck:
- well-defined round hypoechoic lesion within the left parotid;
- it is of homogenous texture and reflectivity with posterior acoustic enhancement, suggesting a solid nature.

MRI of the neck (T1 coronal, STIR coronal, axial proton density):
- solitary, unilateral, well-defined mass lesion within the superficial portion of the left parotid;
- this is of homogenous high signal on T2-weighted images, intermediate signal on T1-weighted images (isointense to muscle) and intermediate signal on T1 fat-suppressed images;
- no cervical lymphadenopathy;
- the right parotid has a normal appearance.

Main diagnosis
In view of the hypoechoic ultrasound appearances and bright T2 signal and intermediate T1 signal on MRI, as well as the fact that the lesion is solitary, and the patient is a middle-aged female, a pleomorphic adenoma is the most likely diagnosis.

Differential diagnoses
A Warthin's tumour could have a similar appearance but a more heterogeneous signal on T2 would be more usual.

Further management
- Fine needle aspiration cytology under ultrasound guidance
- If any diagnostic doubt, post-contrast MRI would be helpful to look for avid enhancement

Discussion
Painless masses in the salivary glands are usually due to a neoplasm, cyst or lymph node, whereas painful masses may be caused by obstructive or inflammatory pathology. In adults, generally, the larger the gland, the lower the frequency of malignancy in mass lesions. However, in the parotid, clinical signs of malignancy include a dull pain, infiltration of the overlying skin, regional adenopathy or facial nerve palsy. In the parotid gland, 80% of tumours are benign, and 80% of those are pleomorphic adenomas. Most (80%) of these occur in the superficial lobe and 80% of untreated adenomas remain benign, with a small proportion undergoing malignant change.

Pleomorphic adenomas are also known as benign mixed tumours and occur most frequently in middle-aged females. Ultrasound features include hypoechoic, well-defined, lobulated with posterior acoustic enhancement, and occasional internal calcifications or anechoic areas. Vascularity is variable, with some lesions having poor or absent vascularity and others having increased vascularity. These tend to be hyperintense on T2-weighted imaging (an indication of benignity), and intermediate signal on T1-weighted imaging, with solid enhancement following contrast administration. Differential diagnoses based on non-contrast images include benign cysts (mucous retention cyst, first branchial cleft cyst, ranula, sialocele), which can also have intermediate T1 signal return in the context of haemorrhage, infection or proteinaceous fluid. Post-contrast images can help to distinguish these entities from pleomorphic adenomata, as the cystic lesions would demonstrate peripheral enhancement.

Warthin's tumour is the second most common benign salivary neoplasm and is more common in middle-aged to elderly males. On ultrasound, the appearances are of an oval, hypoechoic, well-defined lesion that contains multiple anechoic areas and has increased vascularity. It is the most common bilateral or multiple salivary gland tumour. On MRI, particularly, on T2-weighted sequences, these lesions have a more heterogeneous appearance than pleomorphic adenomata.

References

Bialek EJ, Jakubowski W, Zajkowski P, *et al.* US of the major salivary glands: anatomy and spatial relationships, pathologic conditions, and pitfalls. *Radiographics.* 2006; **26**(3): 745–63.

Yousem DM, Kraut MA, Chalian AA. Major salivary gland imaging. *Radiology.* 2000; **216**(1): 19–29.

Case F

History

A 70-year-old male patient with symptoms of urinary tract infection

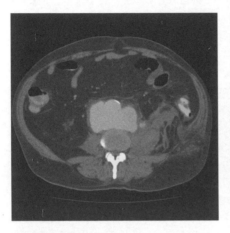

Figure i Arterial phase CT

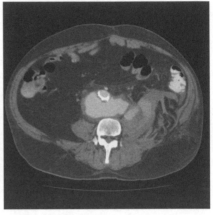

Figure ii Arterial phase CT

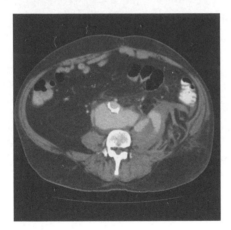

Figure iii Arterial phase CT

Observations and interpretation

Arterial phase CT of the abdomen and pelvis:

- leaking infrarenal aortic aneurysm with haemorrhagic extension into the left psoas;
- haziness of the periaortic fat, suggesting an infected aneurysm;
- the aneurysm does not extend into the iliac arteries;
- small amount of perisplenic free fluid;
- right renal calculus but no evidence of hydronephrosis;
- cystectomy and ileal conduit;
- small liver cyst, with normal solid organs otherwise;
- no lytic or sclerotic bone lesions;
- no mediastinal lymphadenopathy or parenchymal lung lesions.

Main diagnosis

Leaking infected abdominal aortic aneurysm

Differential diagnoses

None

Further management

Urgent referral to Vascular surgeons with a view to emergency surgery

Discussion

Infected aneurysms (also known as mycotic aneurysms) can be complicated by septicaemia, spontaneous rupture and death. The prevalence is approximately 1% and is most common in the aorta, related to intravenous drug use, previous invasive vascular procedure, immunosuppression or chronic illness, including malignancy. The femoral artery is the most commonly involved peripheral artery, usually in the context of intravenous drug abuse. *Staphylococcus* and *Streptococcus* are the often-detected pathogens.

Development of infected aneurysms can arise secondary to:

- haematogenous spread of circulating bacteria
- infection of a pre-existing intimal defect by haematogenous spread
- contiguous spread from an adjacent source
- direct infection of vessel wall from trauma.

The clinical manifestations are diverse and are related to the location of the infected aneurysm. There are usually systemic symptoms of occult infection, with localised features, or, in the more extreme scenario, life-threatening haemorrhage. Infected abdominal aortic aneurysms usually present with abdominal pain, which may be associated with a pulsatile mass. Thoracic aortic aneurysms may present with chest or intrascapular pain. Infected peripheral aneurysms may be associated with a pulsatile mass, pain, palpable thrill, local signs of inflammation, distal emboli or local neurological compression.

Imaging is used to establish the diagnosis, localise and assess the number of aneurysms, identify any complications, plan vascular procedures and surveillance post treatment. CT is generally used initially because of its speed and anatomical accuracy. MRI can be used if the patient is unable to undergo CT angiography or conventional angiography. A T1-weighted fat-suppressed sequence may be helpful to assess the vessel wall and perivascular tissues for abnormal contrast enhancement. Ultrasound is helpful for assessment of peripheral arteries. Nuclear imaging, such as gallium scanning or indium-labelled white cell scans, were used previously but have been replaced by CT. PET-CT may be used for identification of infected aneursysms but has a limited role, in view of the standard non-contrast CT component.

Early signs of aortitis may be identified on CT, which include an irregular arterial wall, peri-aortic oedema (fat stranding or low-density rim), soft tissue mass or gas. CT features of an infected aortic aneurysm include focal, enhancing dilatation that is usually saccular, with a central or eccentric lumen, which may consist of single or multiple compartments. Calcification and thrombus are uncommon. In the context of rupture, haemorrhage may be seen in the pararenal space, perirenal space and peritoneal cavity.

Treatment varies from aggressive antibiotic therapy, to endovascular treatment to surgery, depending on the clinical scenario. However, early diagnosis and aggressive treatment are important to improve prognosis – therefore, it is important to be aware of the imaging features, particularly early signs of arteritis.

Reference
Lee WK, Mossop PJ, Little AF, *et al.* Infected (mycotic) aneurysms: spectrum of imaging appearances and management. *Radiographics*. 2008; **28**(7): 1853–68.

Paper 10

Case A

History

A term neonate with persistent abdominal distention and failure to pass meconium

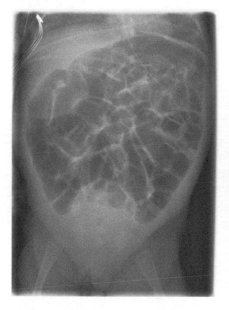

Figure i Abdominal radiograph

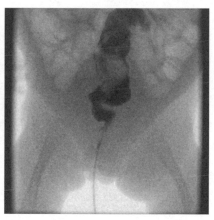

Figure ii Contrast enema

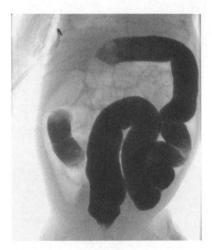

Figure iii Contrast enema

Observations and interpretation

Abdominal radiograph:
- prominent loops of large and small bowel, indicating a low obstruction;
- no gas visible in the rectum;
- no evidence of pneumoperitoneum.

Contrast enema:
- the rectum appears narrower than the adjacent sigmoid colon, consistent with a reversed recto-sigmoid ratio;
- some passive distension of the rectum;
- colon has a slightly increased diameter;
- no filling defects or strictures identified.

Main diagnosis

Functional obstruction – short-segment Hirschsprung's disease

Differential diagnoses

Mechanical obstruction is unlikely, as the rectum passively distends and no stricture or filling defects are appreciated. Potential causes of mechanical obstruction include meconium plug syndrome.

Further management

- Referral to paediatric surgeons; suction mucosal biopsy of the rectum is performed, usually followed by operative management
- Look for other manifestations of a potentially associated syndrome

Discussion

Diagnosis of a gastrointestinal tract anomaly in the neonate or infant relies predominantly on clinical findings. The role of diagnostic imaging is to help determine as accurately as possible the nature of the abnormality. Intestinal obstructions in the neonate are usually classified as high or low and as complete or incomplete.

Hirschsprung's disease is a congenital disorder causing low, usually incomplete, functional colonic obstruction. This is due to an absence of parasympathetic ganglia in the Meissner's and Auberbach's plexuses leading to a hypertonic aganglionic segment of bowel. This can occur at varying distances form the anus but rectosigmoid short segment disease accounts for 80%. Other manifestations include ultra-short segment, long-segment disease, total colonic aganglionosis and skip aganglionosis. It has clinical associations with Down's syndrome and multiple endocrine neoplasia, type II. The majority of patients (up to 80%) present within the first 6 weeks of life and account for up to a quarter of all cases of neonatal bowel obstruction. If identified early then complications of colitis or bowel perforation are rare.

Radiological investigation of choice is a contrast enema without bowel preparation (this can reduce the sensitivity of the study), this study may demonstrate the transition zone between ganglionic and aganglionic segments of bowel. A further strong indicator is a reversed recto-sigmoid ratio – that is, the rectum is smaller than the sigmoid, when it in normal individuals it is the reverse. Other imaging findings include a corrugated rectosigmoid and delayed evacuation of contrast medium. Of note, up to one-third of cases can have a normal appearing enema on fluoroscopy.

Reference

Berrocal T, Lamas M, Gutieérrez J, *et al*. Congenital anomalies of the small intestine, colon, and rectum. *Radiographics*. 1999; **19**(5): 1219–36.

Case B

History

A 30-year-old female with a 1-week history of generalised abdominal pain and diarrhoea

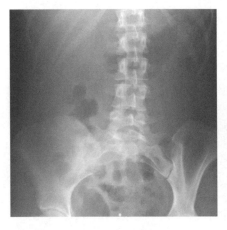

Figure i Abdominal radiograph

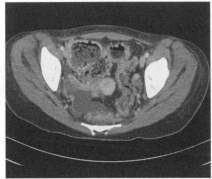

Figure ii Portal venous phase CT

Observations and interpretation

Abdominal radiograph:
- no evidence of organomegaly or pneumoperitoneum;
- suggestion of 'thumbprinting' involving the transverse colon;
- no abnormal calcification;
- unremarkable skeleton.

Portal venous phase CT of the abdomen and pelvis:
- diffuse bowel wall thickening and associated inflammation involving the whole of the colon. This is in keeping with an inflammatory process involving the colon;
- no evidence of colonic obstruction or significant dilatation, although there are several prominent loops;
- the small bowel appears unremarkable;
- no evidence of perforation;
- the liver, gallbladder, biliary tree, pancreas, spleen, adrenals and kidneys are unremarkable – specifically, no gallstones;
- the urinary bladder is catheterised, the pelvic organs are unremarkable;
- moderate amount free fluid in the pelvis;

- no suspicious bony lesions seen, particularly the sacro-iliac joints appear unremarkable;
- lung bases are clear.

Main diagnosis
Pancolitis – most likely secondary to inflammatory bowel disease (the pattern is most in keeping with ulcerative colitis)

Differential diagnoses
- Other colitides:
- Crohn's disease: the contiguous inflammation involving the whole of the colon but sparing the small bowel would be very unusual for Crohn's.
- Pseudomembranous colitis: could give this picture but would be unlikely in a patient of this age. Clinical history (e.g. antibiotic use) and stool cultures would be required for the diagnosis.
- Other infective colitides: as before it would be important to know if the patient was immunocompromised or any other relevant history (e.g. travel).
- Ischaemic colitis: very unlikely in a young patient, it would be unusual to affect the whole of the colon, additionally there is no evidence of arteriopathy.
- Radiation or neutropaenic colitis: this diagnosis would be entirely reliant on the clinical history.

Further management
- Inform the referring team
- Review any previous imaging for supporting features of inflammatory bowel disease
- Suggest low threshold for repeat imaging (e.g. abdominal radiograph) because of risk of toxic megacolon
- Stool cultures should be performed
- Rectal biopsy after the acute episode could be considered to confirm ulcerative colitis

Discussion
Colitis is an umbrella term for inflammation of the colon with different underlying aetiologies. Plain abdominal films can demonstrate bowel wall thickening, potential complications and ancillary findings that may suggest an underlying aetiology. Plain films obviously have a limited sensitivity and

specificity. CT is very commonly utilised in patients with suspected colitis, particularly in the acute setting. CT is excellent at delineating the presence and extent of inflammation, complications and underlying aetiology in many inflammatory conditions of the colon. Distinguishing between the different aetiologies of colitis depends heavily on clinical history and demographic of the patient rather than radiological findings. However, there are obviously certain features that the radiologist can use to favour certain diagnoses.

Inflammatory bowel disease

There may be considerable overlap between the CT findings in Crohn's disease and in ulcerative colitis. However, there are often certain features that may help distinguish the two. Extensive involvement of the right colon and small intestine is more common in Crohn's disease, although involvement of the left colon does occur. In contrast, ulcerative colitis is typically left sided or diffuse (i.e. pancolitis) and only rarely involves the right colon exclusively. At CT, the most frequent finding in both Crohn's disease and ulcerative colitis is wall thickening. The mean wall thickness in Crohn's disease is usually greater than in ulcerative colitis. Wall thickening in ulcerative colitis may be diffuse and symmetric, whereas wall thickening in Crohn's disease is commonly eccentric and segmental with skip regions. The asymmetry of the disease involvement, which typically occurs along the mesenteric border of the intestine, can result in the formation of pseudodiverticula along the antimesenteric border. Pseudodiverticula are small outpouchings of the colonic wall that occur opposite regions of scarring.

Complications of inflammatory bowel disease can also help distinguish between the two pathologies. For example, abscesses and fistulae are detected almost exclusively in Crohn's disease and not in ulcerative colitis.

Infectious colitis

There are many causes of infectious colitis. Bacterial causes include *Shigella*, *Salmonella*, *Yersinia*, *Campylobacter*, *Staphylococcus* and *Chlamydia trachomatis*. Fungal infections such as histoplasmosis, mucormycosis and actinomycosis can affect the colon. Viral causes of colitis include herpesvirus, cytomegalovirus, and rotavirus. Amebiasis and tuberculosis can also cause a colitis, which can resemble inflammatory bowel disease. In general, the infectious colitides are typically diagnosed clinically and do not require CT for detection or differential diagnosis. However, they may be identified at CT incidentally or in cases in which the clinical symptoms are not straightforward.

Many findings are non-specific, therefore clinical history and laboratory studies are necessary for definitive diagnosis. The portion of colon affected may suggest a specific organism. For instance, most cases of infectious colitis are limited to the right colon (*Shigella*, *Salmonella*), although diffuse involvement also occurs (cytomegalovirus, *Escherichia coli*). In contrast, gonorrhea, herpes virus, and *C. trachomatis* (lymphogranuloma venereum) typically involve the rectosigmoid.

Pseudomembranous colitis

Pseudomembranous colitis results from toxins produced by an overgrowth of the organism *Clostridium difficile*. The diagnosis is typically made with stool analysis. Early diagnosis is important as if not treated aggressively it can result in significant morbidity and mortality. At CT, the wall thickening in pseudomembranous colitis is often irregular and shaggy. The target sign is occasionally seen in pseudomembranous colitis. When haustral folds are significantly thickened, they can appear as broad transverse bands that may trap oral contrast material. This appearance is known as the accordion sign. The accordion sign is very suggestive of pseudomembranous colitis but typically occurs only in severe cases and is therefore not a sensitive indicator. In its classic form, pseudomembranous colitis is a pancolitis. However, in some cases it may begin in the rectum and progress retrogradely to involve the left colon. It can also be limited to the right side of the colon with sparing of the left colon. The presence of ascites can also indicate pseudomembranous colitis as the underlying aetiology.

Ischaemic colitis

Most patients are elderly and many have a history of heart disease or vasculopathy. Colonic ischaemia can be the result of generalised hypoperfusion or can also result from occlusion of the mesenteric vasculature by a thrombus, embolus or invasive tumour. Both arterial and venous occlusion can result in colonic ischaemia. The extent and severity of the ischaemia vary with its cause and the vessels involved. Watershed areas of the colon (the splenic flexure and rectosigmoid) are particularly susceptible to ischaemia due to hypovolemia. These regions represent areas of relatively poor perfusion at the border of major vascular territories. Although left-sided involvement is typical in elderly patients with hypoperfusion, right-sided colonic ischaemia and necrosis has been reported in patients as a complication of haemorrhagic shock in trauma.

In patients with colonic ischaemia, CT findings are often non-specific and the diagnosis may be challenging. Clinical correlation is usually required for diagnosis.

Diverticulitis

At CT diverticulitis appears as segmental wall thickening and hyperaemia with inflammatory changes in the pericolic fat. The key to distinguishing diverticulitis from other inflammatory conditions that affect the colon is the presence of diverticula in the involved segment. Also, diverticulitis typically occurs in the descending or sigmoid colon.

Typhlitis

Typhlitis or neutropenic enterocolitis, occurs in neutropenic patients usually undergoing chemotherapy. Typhlitis is characterised by oedema and inflammation of the caecum, the ascending colon and sometimes the terminal ileum.

Radiation colitis

Radiation therapy can result in injury to the colon. Acute radiation injury to the small intestine and colon occurs during or within a few weeks of radiation exposure.

Graft-versus-host disease

Graft-versus-host disease is a complication of allogeneic bone marrow transplantation that occurs when the donor lymphocytes in the graft mount an immunologic attack against the host. The skin, liver and gastrointestinal tract (predominantly the ileum and colon) are the primary organs affected.

References

Thoeni RF, Cello JP. CT imaging of colitis. *Radiology*. 2006; **240**(3): 623–38.

Horton KM, Corl FM, Fishman EK. CT evaluation of the colon: inflammatory disease. *Radiographics*. 2000; **20**(2): 399–418.

Case C

History

Right flank pain, impaired renal function

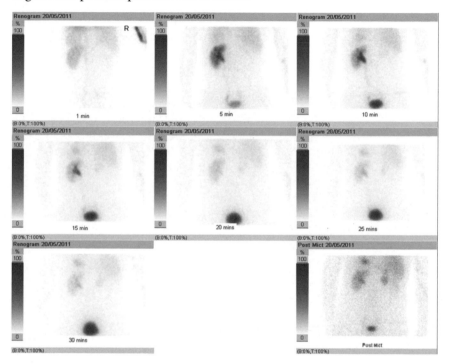

Figure i Nuclear medicine renogram MAG3

185

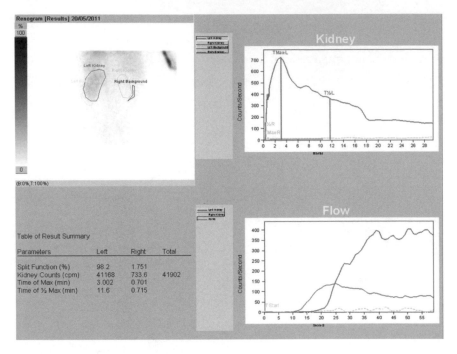

Figure ii Nuclear medicine renogram MAG3

Observations and interpretation

Nuclear medicine renogram MAG3:
- the right kidney is non-functioning;
- the left is appropriately hypertrophied and functioning normally;
- the time activity curves show a normal vascular phase on the left with no evidence of delayed excretion.

Main diagnosis
Non-functioning right kidney

Differential diagnoses
Congenitally absent right kidney (assuming that a previous nephrectomy would be known about)

Further management
- Referral to the appropriate Urological MDT meeting
- Consider performing an ultrasound of the renal tract in the first instance to determine presence of kidney, size, morphology and signs of obstruction

Discussion
Renal radionuclide imaging has always been an important part of renal imaging due to the ability to assess functional parameters. Radiopharmaceuticals are well suited for evaluating blood flow, nephron function, nephron mass, collecting system excretory function and drainage.

MAG3 studies give very useful dynamic information. MAG3 is an acronym for mercaptoacetyltriglycine, a compound that is chelated with technetium-99m. These studies give highly accurate estimated renal plasma flow and good cortical detail.

In dynamic imaging, there are several phases that require characterisation. The first is the flow phase which assesses arterial flow and occurs in the first minute post injection. The next phase is uptake or cortical phase, which occurs until radiotracer begins to leave the parenchyma 3–4 minutes post injection. The excretory phase begins after the uptake phase although both continue to occur simultaneously. The excretory phase is used to assess the collecting system and ureters; excretion is normally plotted on a graph where assessment can be made to identify delayed excretion or obstruction. Differential function is routinely calculated and is obtained by drawing regions of interest then using subtraction calculations.

In this case it is clear that the right kidney is non-functioning, the causes of this are multiple and diverse. These include the following.
- Absence of the kidney:
  - agenesis
  - nephrectomy
  - ectopic kidney
- Loss of perfusion:
  - Infarction – arterial or venous

- Trauma
- Chronic obstructive uropathy:
  - PUJO
  - urethral stricture
  - malignant cause
- Replaced renal parenchyma:
  - multicystic kidney disease
  - tumour
  - infection

Imaging (ultrasound, CT or MRI) will help differentiate between these pathologies in a *de novo* presentation. More than one modality may be utilised; for instance, if ultrasound identifies a severely atrophic kidney then MRI or CT angiography may be used to identify vasculopathy as the cause. Appropriate investigations very much depend on the clinical context.

Reference

Durand E, Chaumet-Riffaud P, Grenier N. Functional renal imaging: new trends in radiology and nuclear medicine. *Semin Nucl Med.* 2011; **41**(1): 61–72.

Case D

History

A 16-year-old with painful hips for 1 week

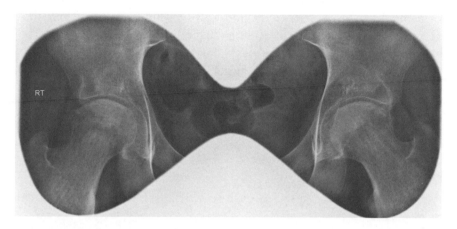

Figure i Pelvic radiograph

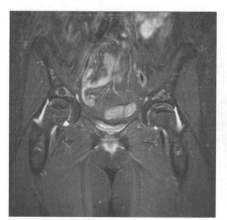

Figure ii Coronal T1 MRI

Figure iii Coronal STIR MRI

Observations and interpretation

Radiograph of the pelvis (coned view)

- there is irregularity of the femoral heads, with sclerosis and subchondral lucency.

MRI of the pelvis (T1 and STIR coronal)

- the coronal T1-weighted sequences demonstrate low signal subchrondal curvilinear lines within the femoral heads, which is consistent with avascular necrosis;
- the fluid sensitive sequences demonstrate curvilinear high signal in the femoral head subchondral region on the left;
- small bilateral joint effusions;
- in addition, there are a number of well-defined areas with low signal borders throughout the bony pelvis and proximal femora, in keeping with bone infarcts or multifocal osteonecrosis;
- bone infarcts are also noted in the L5 and S1 vertebral bodies;
- no extraosseous abnormalities.

Main diagnosis

Avascular necrosis of the femoral heads bilaterally with multifocal involvement

Differential diagnoses

None

Further management

Urgent discussion with the referring clinicians

Discussion

In this case, the patient was being treated for an underlying malignancy with steroids (although there are a large number of aetiologies for these appearances, sickle cell would also be a possibility in this age group). The epiphysis and metaphysis of long tubular bones are at risk of osteonecrosis because of a limited arterial supply and limited venous drainage.

Avascular necrosis (AVN) is due to insufficient perfusion in the articular ends of bones, where a balance of necrosis and repair occurs. Reactive new bone forms over dead trabeculae, which leads to a sclerotic appearance. Mechanical failure occurs at the interface of necrosis and repair, which leads to micofracture and collapse of the adjacent dead subchondral trabeculae. This appears as a subchondral radiolucency, described as the crescent sign. Subsequently, there is collapse of the femoral head on the articular surface, which is associated with cartilage destruction and premature osteoarthritis.

There are four clinical and radiographic stages of AVN, based on the Ficat classification system. In stage 1, the plain radiograph appears normal, but the MRI or radionuclide bone scan is abnormal, confirming AVN. Cystic and sclerotic changes are seen on the radiographs in stage 2. The crescent sign is seen in stage 3. Stage 4 consists of flattening of the femoral head, hip joint narrowing and joint destruction. (There is also a stage 0 in a modified classification, which is when the patient is suspected of having AVN without clinical or radiographic findings.) MRI and radionuclide imaging are useful for risk stratification and planning the appropriate timing of head-preserving surgeries. MRI is particularly useful in the early diagnosis of AVN, with a reported sensitivity of 97% and specificity of 98%. MRI is particularly useful in the diagnosis of early marrow oedema.

Another sign that is seen with AVN, is the double line sign, which is observed on T2-weighted images of medullary bone as a high-signal intensity line with a parallel rim of decreased signal intensity. The high-signal inner zone represents hyperemic granulation tissue at the interface between necrosis and repair. The low-signal outer zone reflects sclerotic bone.

References

Pappas JN. The musculoskeletal crescent sign. *Radiology*. 2000; **217**(1): 213–14.
Zurlo JV. The double-line sign. *Radiology*. 1999; **212**(2): 541–2.

Case E
History
A 50-year-old female patient, confused

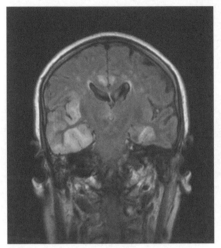

Figure i Coronal fluid-attenuated inversion recovery MRI

Figure ii Axial proton density MRI

Observations and interpretation
MRI of the brain (axial proton density, coronal fluid-attenuated inversion recovery (FLAIR) and diffusion-weighted imaging):
- asymmetric bilateral high T2 and FLAIR signal in the anterior and medial temporal lobes bilaterally, extending into the insula on the right, with local sulcal effacement;
- high signal intensity on diffusion-weighted imaging (DWI) but not apparent diffusion coefficient (ADC) within both the insula and right anterior temporal lobe reflects oedema rather than infarct;
- no evidence of midline shift;
- the ventricles are normal size and configuration;
- high T2 signal foci in the centrum semiovale reflects background white matter disease.

Main diagnosis
Herpes simplex encephalitis

Differential diagnoses
Other viral encephalitides

Further management

Refer to neurology for antiviral therapy

Discussion

Herpes simplex virus (HSV) encephalitis causes a haemorrhagic, necrotising encephalitis and is the most prevalent viral encephalitis in the developed world. There are severe memory and personality problems in those that survive without treatment. It affects the limbic system, medial temporal lobes and inferior frontal lobes. The oral strain (type 1) and the genital strain (type 2) can cause encephalitis. Type 2 is more common in the neonatal period. The MRI features can be characteristic and can prevent the need for a biopsy.

The clinical symptoms of type 1 HSV encephalitis include acute confusion, disorientation, stupor and coma. There may be a viral prodrome associated with seizures. Left temporal lobe involvement affects language and therefore may become symptomatic earlier. The pathologic features are of asymmetric involvement of the temporal lobes, insula, bifrontal region and cingulate gyrus. One-third are due to primary activation and approximately two-thirds from reactivation.

On CT, the appearances of HSV encephalitis include a normal scan if the patient presents early in the disease process, low-attenuation in the temporal lobes, with sparing of the putamen, temporal lobe swelling, haemorrhage, if there is fulminant encephalitis, or contract enhancement of parenchyma or gyri.

MRI features include increased T2 and FLAIR signal of the cerebral cortex, temporal lobe, insula and cingulate gyrus. This appearance may be of asymmetric bilateral abnormalities. The diffusion-weighted pattern may be positive or negative. Negative diffusion may reflect potential for reversibility. Other features are gyral enhancement, haemorrhage (high T1 signal on the pre-contrast images), atrophy and encephalomalacia. Mass effect from temporal lobe oedema may persist for a number of weeks. If untreated, there is a 70% mortality rate – therefore, it is important to consider this differential and recommend MRI.

References

Chapman S, Nakielny R. *Aids to Radiological Differential Diagnosis*. 4th ed. Edinburgh: Saunders, Elsevier; 2007.

Grossman RI, Yousem DM. *Neuroradiology: The Requisites*. 2nd ed. Philadelphia, USA: Mosby; 2003.

Case F

History

A 5-year-old with general malaise

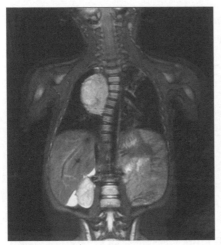

Figure i MRI coronal T1 FS

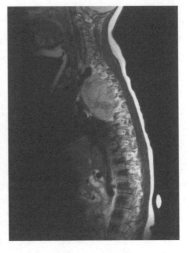

Figure ii MRI sagittal T2

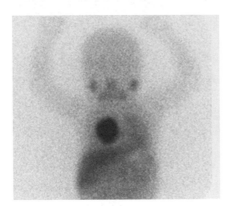

Figure iii MIBG scan

Observations and interpretation

MRI of the chest (T1 fat-saturated coronal, T2 axil, sagittal and coronal):

- low T1 signal mass within the posterior mediastinum;
- the mass is high signal on STIR and intermediate signal on T2;
- low-signal areas that reflect calcification;
- the mass crosses the midline and is close to the descending thoracic aorta;
- the mass extends below the carina, displaces the right main bronchus and encases the left main bronchus;
- collapse of the left upper lobe apical segment.

MIBG scan:

- there is an intense focus of activity within the chest but no distant disease.

Main diagnosis

Neuroblastoma within the posterior mediastinum

Differential diagnoses

None

Further management

Further to Paediatric surgeons and discussion at the Paediatric Oncology MDT meeting

Discussion

It is important to assess the various lines in the chest in the diagnosis of a mediastinal mass. Features in the assessment of a posterior mediastinal mass include disruption of the azygo-oesophgeal recess, disruption of the paraspinal lines and visualisation of masses above the clavicles.

The differential for posterior mediastinal masses includes oesophageal lesions, foregut duplication cysts, descending aortic aneurysms, neurogenic tumours (neurofibroma/schwannoma), paraspinal abscess, lateral meningocele and extramedullary haematopoiesis. CT is generally used as the next investigation, which confirms the position of the mass and helps to characterise the mass further. MRI is used for neurogenic tumours, providing a greater degree of information regarding spinal involvement.

Neuroblastomas are a malignancy of the sympathetic nervous system and belong to the group of tumours known as neuroblastic tumours. Neuroblastoma is the most immature, undifferentiated and malignant tumour of the neuroblastic group. This accounts for 10% of paediatric tumours and 15% of cancer deaths in children. The clinical presentation is usually of pain due to either local mass effect or metastatic disease. Other signs include fatigue, malaise, weight loss, shortness of breath (if abdominal primary) or neurology (if involving nerve roots or spinal canal). There is an international neuroblastoma staging system, ranging from stage 1 (localised tumour at area of origin) to stage 4 (dissemination to nodes, bone, liver or other organs) or stage 4S (localised primary with disseminated disease in patients under 1 year).

Radiographs may show a soft tissue mass, with calcification in 30% of cases. Ultrasound shows a heterogeneous appearance and may be useful for evaluation of metastatic disease. CT is the most useful modality to assess extent of primary, organ of origin, regional invasion, vascular encasement, adenopathy, calcification and distant disease. MRI appearances are of heterogeneous, low T1 and high T2 signal areas, with variable enhancement. MRI is helpful in assessment of intraspinal extension. Nuclear medicine is useful for identification of the primary and for surveillance using MIBG (metaiodobenzylguanidine labelled to iodine-123). Bone scintigraphy can also be helpful in assessment of bone metastases. The most important prognostic indicators are age of patient at diagnosis and stage of disease.

References
Kawashima A, Fishman EK, Kuhlman JE, *et al.* CT of posterior mediastinal masses. *Radiographics.* 1991; **11**(6): 1045–67.

Lonergan GJ, Schwab CM, Suarez ES, *et al.* Neuroblastoma, ganglioneuroblastoma and ganglioneuroma: radiologic-pathologic correlation. *Radiographics.* 2002; **22**(4): 911–34.

Whitten CR, Khan S, Munneke GJ, *et al.* A diagnostic approach to mediastinal abnormalities. *Radiographics.* 2007; **27**(3): 657–71.

Paper 11

Case A
History
A child with asthma and productive cough with subsequent development of leg weakness and altered sensation

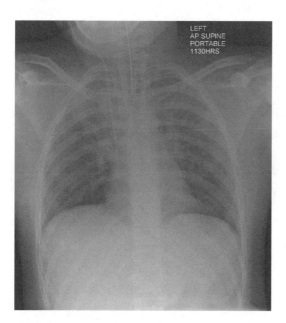

Figure i Chest radiograph

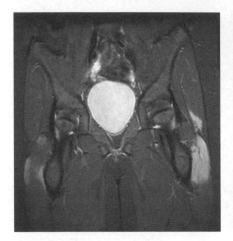 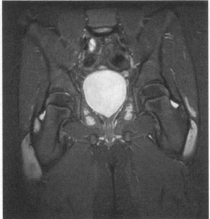

Figure ii Coronal STIR MRI   **Figure iii** Coronal STIR MRI

Observations and interpretation

Chest radiograph

- appropriately placed endotracheal tube tip, right internal jugular central line and nasogastric tube;
- cardiac contours within normal size limits;
- increased opacification particularly prominent in the right upper lobe and to a milder degree in the left upper lobe in keeping with atelectasis;
- no evidence of pleural effusion or pneumothorax.

MRI of the pelvis (T1 coronal, axial proton density, STIR coronal):

- abnormal signal intensity is seen arising from the vastus lateralis muscles bilaterally;
- this involves the proximal muscles towards their insertions with less marked involvement of the glutei;
- this fluid signal demonstrates oedema and is most in keeping with an inflammatory process;
- normal signal return from the bones;
- the course of the sciatic nerves is unremarkable;
- no neural abnormality.

Main diagnosis

Post-infectious polymyositis following a lower respiratory tract infection/ infective exacerbation of asthma

Differential diagnoses
None

Further management
Referral to Paediatricians for further management (including steroids plus or minus immunotherapy)

Discussion
Polymyositis is an inflammatory autoimmune disorder causing proximal muscle weakness and muscular pain, usually of insidious onset. When it occurs in conjunction with a characteristic exanthma (rash) it is termed dermatomyositis. In the paediatric population, it is most commonly seen following an infective process but in older patients, it is often a paraneoplastic phenomenon, associated with an underlying neoplasia. Of note, it can also be a manifestation of HIV/AIDS in both the adult and paediatric populations.

The underlying pathophysiology is a cell-mediated/type IV autoimmune response. Diagnosis is usually by a combination of clinical history, raised creatine kinase and autoantibodies, as well as radiology. Muscle biopsy is occasional performed if there is uncertainty over the diagnosis.

When involving skeletal muscle, the thigh (particularly the vastus lateralis and intermedius muscles), is the site affected most frequently. Acutely, it causes bilateral, symmetrical oedema within the muscle. In more chronic episodes, there can also be fatty infiltration and muscle atrophy. Eventually sheet-like confluent calcifications in the soft tissues of the extremities characterises this condition. The initial imaging may be helpful to guide muscle biopsy.

Other involved systems include skeletal (arthropathy and resorption of the terminal tufts of the phalanges), respiratory (muscle weakness, fibrosis and bronchiolitis obliterans organising pneumonia), myocardial (myopathy) and gastrointestinal (dysphagia and atony of smooth muscle).

Immunosuppression forms the mainstay of treatment, with follow-up guided by clinical response and muscle enzyme levels. Complications include those from steroid therapy and those from the myositis (aspiration pneumonia, myocardial infarction, interstitial lung disease, dysphagia).

Reference
Stiglbauer R, Graninger W, Prayer L, *et al*. Polymyositis: MRI-appearance at 1.5 T and correlation to clinical findings. *Clin Radiol*. 1993; **48**(4): 244–8.

Case B

History

A 33-year-old female of West African origin, presenting with a 4-day history of fever and right upper quadrant pain

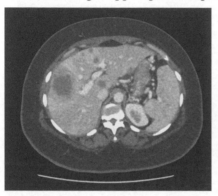

Figure i Portal venous phase CT

Figure ii Portal venous phase CT

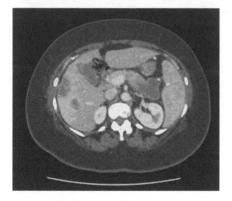

Figure iii Portal venous phase CT

Observations and interpretation

Portal venous phase CT of the abdomen and pelvis:

- liver is grossly abnormal with geographic enhancement and multiple target type lesions in both lobes;
- most of these lesions have necrotic centres with a thick circumferential wall – these cystic lesions could be inflammatory or malignant in nature;
- gallbladder is thin walled with no stones seen;
- neck, head and uncinate process of the pancreas is normal but the tail and distal body enhances poorly;

- this area appears diffusely enlarged with stranding in the surrounding fat – again, this could be an inflammatory or malignant process;
- no pancreatic duct dilatation;
- enlarged precaval nodes;
- normal spleen, adrenals and kidneys;
- bowel loops are unremarkable but there is close relation of the splenic flexure to the pancreatic tail;
- small volume of free fluid in the pelvis;
- no suspicious bony lesions;
- bibasal atelectasis.

Main diagnosis

Focal pancreatitis with hepatic abscesses: this would seem most likely in a young patient with a history of fever

Differential diagnoses

- Pancreatic carcinoma with necrotic hepatic metastases: although radiologically this could be the principle diagnosis, the age and history of the patient somewhat favour an inflammatory process. Fever, however, can be associated with malignancy. Additionally cystic metastases are atypical for pancreatic adenocarcinoma.
- Atypical lymphoma: lymphoma has a myriad of radiological appearances and should be considered but the liver lesions in particular are atypical and there is no splenomegaly.
- Hepatic and pancreatic metastases from an unidentified primary: this appearance of the pancreatic pathology is atypical for pancreatic metastases but this should be considered.
- Dual unrelated pathology – for example, pancreatic tumour and hepatic abscesses (e.g. amoebic, mycobacterial or other infective abscesses)

Further management

- For discussion at Gastrointestinal MDT meeting
- Inform referring team of findings
- Consider ultrasound of the liver to further characterise hepatic lesions and potentially procede to aspiration/biopsy
- Consider MRI liver to further characterise lesions
- If confirmed hepatic abscesses, interventional radiologist may insert drains under image guidance
- Ascertain immune status of patient
- Perform tumour markers

Discussion

The combination of the multiple partially cystic lesions in the liver and the low-attenuation lesion in the pancreas obviously favours certain pathologies, although co-existing but separate aetiologies should always be considered.

The most likely differential diagnoses are liver abscesses associated with a focal pancreatitis or cystic/necrotic metastases from a pancreatic malignancy. In this case the former is considered the most likely, primarily because of the patient's age and the presence of fever. Further clinical information could obviously sway this one way or another.

This is a difficult case to discuss in full and further reading may be necessary. For the sake of the discussion we will look separately at solid pancreatic lesions and cystic lesion of the liver.

Solid lesions of the pancreas represent a heterogeneous group of entities that can be broadly classified as either neoplastic or non-neoplastic. Neoplastic lesions include pancreatic adenocarcinoma, pancreatic neuroendocrine tumour, solid pseudopapillary tumour, pancreatoblastoma, pancreatic lymphoma, metastases to the pancreas and rare miscellaneous neoplasms. Non-neoplastic lesions include focal pancreatitis, fatty infiltration/replacement, intrapancreatic accessory spleen, congenital anomalies such as prominent pancreatic lobulation and bifid pancreatic tail (pancreatic bifidum), and rare miscellaneous lesions (e.g. pancreatic sarcoidosis, Castleman's disease of the pancreas).

Equally, the aetiology of cystic lesions of the liver are manifold. Metastases to the liver are common, and a variety of often non-specific appearances have been reported. Most hepatic metastases are solid, but some have a complete or partially cystic appearance. In general, three different pathologic mechanisms can explain the cyst-like appearance of hepatic metastases. First, hypervascular metastatic tumours with rapid growth may lead to necrosis and cystic degeneration, frequently demonstrated in metastases from neuroendocrine tumours, sarcoma, melanoma and certain subtypes of lung and breast carcinoma. Contrast-enhanced CT and MRI typically demonstrate multiple lesions with strong enhancement of the peripheral viable and irregularly defined tissue. Second, cystic metastases may also be seen with mucinous adenocarcinomas, such as colorectal or ovarian carcinoma. Ovarian metastases can often be seen as cystic serosal implants on both the visceral peritoneal surface of the liver and the parietal peritoneum of the diaphragm. This appearance is in contradistinction to that of most other cystic hepatic lesions, which are intraparenchymal. Additionally, solid metastases can become cystic following treatment and subsequent treatment-related necrosis.

Cystic subtypes of primary liver neoplasms are rare and are usually related to internal necrosis following disproportionate growth or systemic and locoregional treatment. Hepatocellular carcinoma and giant cavernous hemangioma are the two most common primary neoplasms of the liver; these rarely manifest as an entirely or partially cystic mass.

Abscesses can be singular but are usually multiple. They can be classified as pyogenic, amoebic or fungal. Pyogenic hepatic abscesses are most commonly caused by *Clostridium* species and Gram-negative bacteria, such as *Escherichia coli* and *Bacteroides* species, which enter the liver via the portal venous system or biliary tree. Ascending cholangitis and portal phlebitis are the most frequent causes of pyogenic hepatic abscesses but they can be associated with haematogenous spread from sepsis anywhere in the body, particularly sites draining into the portal system (e.g. diverticulitis). The overall appearance of a hepatic abscess at cross-sectional imaging varies according to the pathologic stage of the infection. However, they usually appear as thick-walled lesions with central homogeneous low attenuation at CT or fluid signal on MRI. In addition to the enhancing abscess wall, contrast-enhanced CT and especially contrast-enhanced MRI typically show increased peripheral rim enhancement, which is secondary to increased capillary permeability. This creates the (the 'double target' sign). Perilesional oedema is most markedly demonstrated in abscess but is not specific to inflammatory processes and can be seen surrounding malignant deposits. However, the presence of perilesional oedema can be used to differentiate a hepatic abscess from a benign cystic hepatic lesion.

Miscellaneous lesions include hepatic extrapancreatic pseudocysts. Although pancreatic pseudocysts can form anywhere in the abdomen, intrahepatic occurrence is rare. They occur predominantly in the left lobe of the liver, as a result of extension of fluid from the lesser sac into the leaves of the hepatogastric ligament. Clinical symptoms are usually related to the underlying inflammatory pancreatic disease. Elevated serum and urinary amylase levels should arouse suspicion for this condition. Correct diagnosis is not difficult with imaging when other signs of acute pancreatitis are present.

References

Low G, Panu A, Millo N, *et al.* Multimodality imaging of neoplastic and non-neoplastic solid lesions of the pancreas. *Radiographics*. 2011; **31**(4): 993–1015.

Mortelé KJ, Ros PR. Cystic focal liver lesions in the adult: differential CT and MR imaging features. *Radiographics*. 2001; **21**(4): 895–910.

Case C

History

A 45-year-old female undergoing routine breast screening

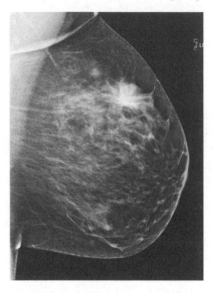

Figure i Left medial-lateral oblique (MLO) mammogram

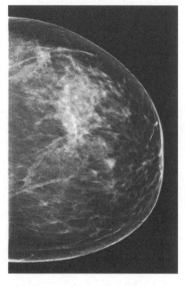

Figure ii Left craniocaudal (CC) mammogram

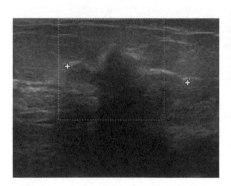

Figure iii Ultrasound of the breast, upper outer quadrant

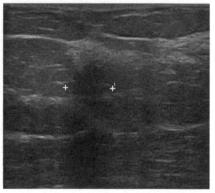

Figure iv Ultrasound of the breast, upper outer quadrant

Observations and interpretation

Mammogram:

- the right breast appears normal;
- on the left side there is a spiculate mass just above and slightly medial to the nipple;
- adjacent to the larger lesion is a further suspicious density on the mammogram.

Ultrasound of the left breast:

- at least two suspicious lesions in the same quadrant of the breast;
- these lesions are ill-defined, are taller than they are wide, have angular margins with normal tissue and cast a posterior acoustic shadow.

Main diagnosis

Multifocal/multicentric carcinoma of the breast

Differential diagnoses

Benign disease mimicking malignant disease, although these lesions are malignant until proven otherwise

Further management

- Urgent referral to Breast clinic and discussion at the MDT meeting
- If appropriate, perform separate core biopsies of the lesions under ultrasound guidance and perform ultrasound assessment of the axilla
- Consider contrast enhanced MRI breasts because of risk in contralateral breast of multifocal disease

Discussion

Mammography is used both in the screening and in the symptomatic setting. An abnormal density on mammography has to be carefully evaluated. A malignancy is suspected if the opacity is spiculated or has a comet tail; other suspicious features include disrupted surrounding parenchyma, retracted or thickened skin, focal dilatation of ducts and certain types of microcalcification. Suspicious features of microcalcification are varied: segmental or cluster distribution, mixture of size and shapes, eccentrically located within a lesion and deterioration on serial mammography. When a lesion is identified on mammography, usually the lesion is further characterised by focal ultrasound.

Ultrasound is very useful in assessing breast disease. The most important task is to differentiate between benign and malignant disease. Typical appearances of a carcinoma on ultrasound include a poorly reflective ill-defined mass, the lesion being taller than it is wide, heterogeneous echogenicity, an angular margin between the abnormal and normal issue, microlobulation, absent 'far wall' echoes and posterior acoustic shadowing. There are obviously plenty of features that suggest benignity but a single malignant feature prohibits classification of a lesion as benign.

There are some benign pathologies that can mimic malignancy on mammography, ultrasound or both – for example, an ill-defined microadenoma, fibromatosis, fat necrosis, sclerosing adenosis, post-procedural scar or haematoma, radial scar, mastitis or abscess and some skin lesions. Of note, a radial scar increases the risk of a subsequent cancer, particularly if this contains hyperplasia, therefore excision is now generally recommended.

Dynamic contrast material-enhanced MRI of the breast is increasingly used as an adjunct to mammography and ultrasound to improve the detection and characterisation of primary and recurrent breast cancers and for evaluation of the response to therapy. MRI is useful for detecting multifocality and multicentricity of breast cancer; differentiating between scar tissue and recurrent cancer after breast-conserving therapy, screening patients in high-risk groups (e.g. those with the BRCA1 gene) and examining breasts that contain implants; examining the breasts of patients with histologically proved metastatic breast cancer with unknown primary origin; and, in patients with a finding of cancer in one breast, screening the contralateral breast for occult cancer. The sensitivity of MRI for the detection of breast cancer is very high.

Failure to diagnose multifocal and multicentric breast cancers can directly affect patient treatment. Multifocal breast cancer is defined as two or more cancers in the same quadrant, whereas multicentric breast cancer is defined as two or more cancers in different quadrants. In multicentric disease, breast conservation therapy is contraindicated. These disease entities may not be perceived owing to 'satisfaction of search'. Careful attention must also be paid to the contralateral breast after observation of suspect lesions because contralateral synchronous cancers are well documented.

All clinical, radiological (regardless of modality) and histological findings are classified by BI-RADS (Breast Imaging-Reporting and Data System) classification.

The BI-RADS assessment categories are:

0 – Incomplete
1 – Negative
2 – Benign findings
3 – Probably benign

4 – Suspicious abnormality
5 – Highly suspicious of malignancy
6 – Known biopsy with proven malignancy categories

Reference

Wilkinson LS, Given-Wilson R, Hall T, *et al.* Increasing the diagnosis of multifocal primary breast cancer by the use of bilateral whole-breast ultrasound. *Clin Radiol.* 2005; **60**(5): 573–8.

Case D

History

A 70-year-old, presented with pain at the right arm after fall

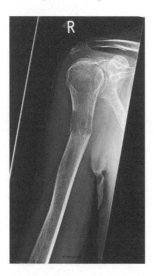

Figure i Radiograph of the right humerus

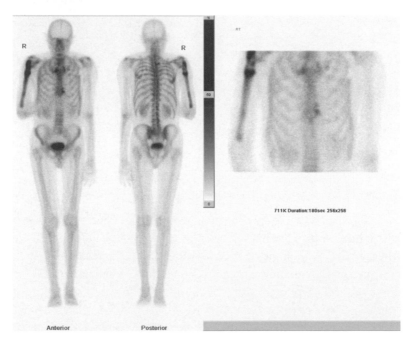

Figure ii Delayed phase bone scan

Observations and interpretation

Radiograph of the right humerus:
- lytic lesion in the proximal humeral shaft, with ill-defined margins, in keeping with an aggressive lesion;
- thinning of the cortex and a pathological fracture;
- no focal lung lesions or other bone lesions.

Delayed phase bone scan:
- high-grade uptake at the right humerus with uptake seen along the length of the right humerus, in keeping with malignant infiltration;
- further uptake at the right posterior fourth rib which is probably also involved;
- uptake at the sternoclavicular joints is probably degenerative.

Main diagnosis

Pathological fracture through lytic deposit, most likely a metastasis, from bronchial, renal, colorectal primary

Differential diagnoses

The differential diagnoses would include myeloma, lymphoma, and primary bone neoplasia, such as an osteosarcoma or chondrosarcoma, although these latter pathologies are less likely.

Further management

- In view of the fracture, an urgent orthopaedic referral is required for fixation.
- To identify the primary lesion, further imaging is required, starting with a chest radiograph and abdominal ultrasound. CT may also be required.

Discussion

Renal cell carcinoma (RCC) typically metastasizes to bone with expansile, purely lytic lesions, which are highly vascular with an associated soft tissue mass. Other primary pathologies that have lytic expansile metastases include those from thyroid malignancy, phaeochromocytoma and melanoma.

It is not uncommon for a clinically occult RCC to manifest as a solitary bone metastasis. Osseous metastases from RCC can occur years later, even if the patient undergoes a nephrectomy, as happens in between 20% and 60% of patients. As with any aggressive bone lesions, in these cases pathological fractures and cord compression may be the presenting features in this patient group. Osseous metastases usually occur in the first few years after resection of the primary tumour, although they can occur up to 20 years later.

There are no pathognomic features of osseous metastases specifically from RCC; however, because of the hypervascular nature of these lesions, the presence of flow voids on MRI has been described. It is important to note that there are a number of primary musculoskeletal and soft tissue lesions that also demonstrate flow voids, including haemangioma, sarcoma subtypes, aneurismal bone cysts and giant cell tumours.

In the context of an osseous metastasis, it is important to consider imaging (either ultrasound or CT chest, abdomen and pelvis) to look for an occult primary lesion, or review the past medical history. Local treatment for these lesions includes surgery, radiotherapy or percutaneous transcatheter arterial embolisation, all of which relieve pain, prevent pathological fractures and improve function and mobility.

References

Chapman S, Nakielny R. *Aids to Radiological Differential Diagnosis*. 4th ed. UK: Saunders, Elsevier; 2007.

Choi JA, Lee KH, Yi MG, *et al.* Osseous metastasis from renal cell carcinoma: 'flow-void' sign at MR imaging. *Radiology*. 2003; **228**(3): 629–34.

Case E

History
A 62-year-old male, 4 days post abdominal surgery

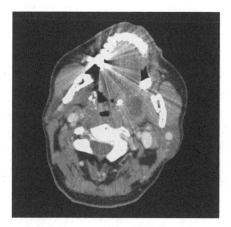

Figure i Arterial phase CT

Observations and interpretation
Arterial phase CT of the neck:
- fluid density, multi-loculated collection at the left tonsillar bed, which extends superiorly towards the tongue base and is suspicious for an abscess;
- peripheral enhancement of the wall and septae, which are of varying thickness;
- this abnormal area extends into the left parapharyngeal space and causes local mass effect and displacement of the oropharynx;
- punctate calcification in the tonsillar bed bilaterally;
- no evidence of collection at the retropharyngeal or prevertebral spaces;
- the left internal jugular vein enhances normally;
- small nodes at levels 2 and 5, consistent with reactive nodes;
- no abnormalities of the visualised mediastinum or lungs.

Main diagnosis
Infective collection at the left tonsillar bed

Differential diagnoses
None

Further management

Discussion with the referring clinicians regarding previous surgery and further management

Discussion

The tonsils are paired bilateral lymphoid tissue at the lateral wall of the oropharynx. Tonsilloliths can develop, which are small areas of calcareous matter that form in the tonsillar crypts and may grow or coalesce to a large size. These may be incidental, in that patients may be asymptomatic, or may be associated with a persistent throat infection, foul taste or otalgia. They have an appearance of 'rice grains', ovoid homogenous dense opacifications, found more medial than the carotid space, which helps to differentiate from carotid artery calcification.

There are a number of deep compartments in the head and neck, including the mucosal, parapharyngeal, parotid, carotid, masticator, retropharyngeal and prevertebral spaces. There is a variety of pathology that can occur in these areas. Key areas to be aware of in the context of infection are the parapharyngeal and retropharyngeal spaces, as it may be difficult to detect abscess clinically at these locations.

The parapharyngeal space is a triangular, fat-filled space that extends from the skull base to the submandibular gland region. It is surrounded by the carotid space posteriorly, the parotid space laterally, the masticator space anteriorly and the superficial muscosal space medially. It therefore indicates mass effect from any pathology in the adjacent spaces.

The retropharyngeal space is a potential space that lies posterior to the superficial mucosal space and anterior to the prevertebral space. A mass in this location leads to posterior displacement of the prevertebral muscles. There is a connection between the retropharyngeal space and the mediastinum, thus providing a potential route for infection or malignancy to extend into the chest. Infections here may be the result of tonsillitis, dental infection, trauma or systemic infections, such as tuberculosis. Both on CT and MRI, contrast-enhanced images are helpful to determine the extent and presence of an abscess or collection in this area.

Reference

Barakis, JA. Head and neck imaging. In: Brant WE, Helms CA. *Fundamentals of Diagnostic Radiology*. 3rd ed. Philadelphia, USA: Lippincott, Williams & Wilkins; 2007. pp. 241–70.

Case F

History

A 65-year-old male with chest pain

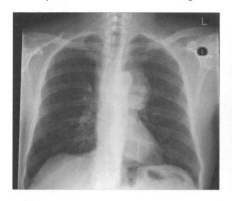

Figure i Chest radiograph

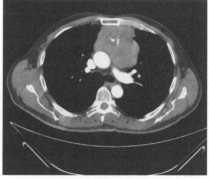

Figure ii Arterial phase CT

Observations and Interpretation

Chest radiograph:

- widening of the superior mediastinum on the left;
- the aortic arch and descending aorta are seen separately, indicating that this mass lies in the anterior mediastinum;
- no evidence of focal lung lesions.

Arterial phase CT of the chest:

- heterogeneous lobulated well-defined mass in the anterior mediastinum;
- the mass demonstrates peripheral enhancement with low attenuation areas;
- irregular calcification in the central part of the mass;
- the fat planes are preserved with no evidence of invasion into vascular structures;
- no evidence of mediastinal lymphadenopathy.

Main diagnosis

Appearances are in keeping with an anterior mediastinal mass. The most likely diagnosis is of a thymic tumour, because of the heterogeneity and calcification.

Differential diagnoses

Teratoma is a further possibility

Further management

Referral to cardiothoracic surgeons for surgical biopsy or excision

Discussion

The anterior mediastinum contains the thymus, lymph nodes, adipose tissue and internal mammary vessels. The thyroid is also considered to be part of the anterior mediastinum if it extends inferiorly. It is important to consider whether there is obliteration of the anterior junction line and presence of the hilum overlay sign. The hilum overlay sign indicates that a mass is either anterior or posterior to the hilum, which is considered to be within the middle mediastinum. Preservation of posterior lines also helps to place an anterior mass.

The typical differential for anterior mediastinal masses includes thyroid tumours, thymoma, teratoma and lymphoma. However, these groups can be subdivided into prevascular, precardiac or other lesions. The prevascular masses include lymphadenopathy, retrosternal goitre and thymic lesions (thymoma, carcinoma, hyperplasia, cysts and thymolipoma). The pre-cardiac masses in contact with the diaphragm include epicardial fat pad, diaphragmatic hump, morgagni herna, pleuropericardial cysts and lymph node enlargement. Rare lesions include lymphatic malformations and haemangiomas.

Reference

Whitten CR, Khan S, Munneke GJ, *et al.* A diagnostic approach to mediastinal abnormalities. *Radiographics.* 2007; **27**(3): 657–71.

Paper 12

Case A
History
A 16-year-old female treated by a general practitioner for recurrent urinary tract infections (UTIs)

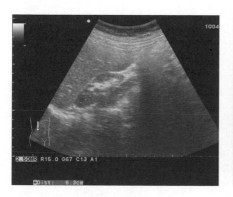

Figure i Ultrasound of the right kidney

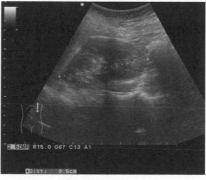

Figure ii Ultrasound of the left kidney

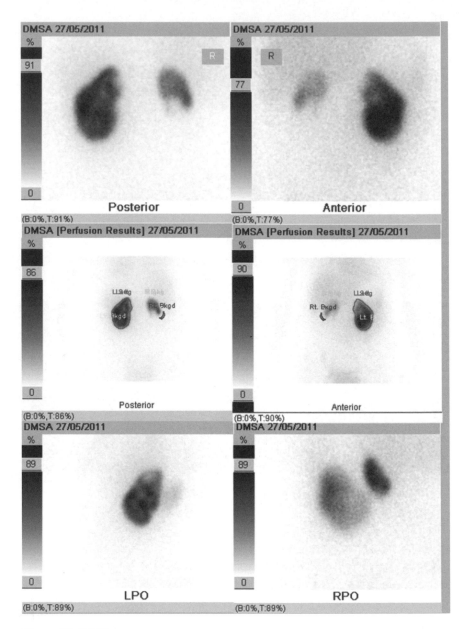

Figure iii DMSA scan

Observations and interpretation

Ultrasound of the urinary tract:

- right kidney is normal in shape but is small with a maximum length of 6.3 cm;

- no upper tract dilatation seen in the right kidney but there is cortical thinning and scarring;
- left kidney appears normal.

Nuclear medicine renal DMSA scan:
- small right kidney contributing only 17% compared with 83% from the left kidney;
- photon deficient area at the lower pole on the right and a smaller photon deficient area at the upper pole on the left;
- appearances suggest bilateral scars.

Main diagnosis
Bilateral renal scarring, more severe on the right – the most common cause would be vesicoureteric reflux

Differential diagnoses
Renal scarring due to a different aetiology – for instance, an underlying structural or functional cause, or recurrent ascending infections without the former

Further management
- Referral to Paediatricians/Renal Physician
- Suggest repeat midstream specimen of urine and antibiotic cover if clinically indicated.
- Consider a micturating cystourogram to investigate possible underlying reflux.

Discussion
The DMSA scan is usually performed with technetium-99m and is excellent for cortical imaging. This gives a more static image of the kidney and assesses cortical binding, which has excellent sensitivity for cortical scarring. If more functional information were required then a MAG3 study would be more suitable as this can assess blood flow, glomerular filtration and tubular secretion together with the structure and function of the collecting systems and ureters. Ureteral reflux can also be assessed by direct radionuclide cystography. This is more sensitive than contrast cystograms, as it can detect very small amounts of reflux.

Primary vesicoureteral reflux (VUR) is the most common congenital urological abnormality in children. Primary VUR has been associated with an increased risk of UTI and renal scarring; it is also called reflux nephropathy (RN). Primary VUR is predominantly caused by a short submucosal tunnel of the distal ureter in the bladder wall, compromising the valvular function. VUR may also occur in the context of an abnormal bladder – that is, secondary to poor bladder emptying – perhaps because of bladder outlet obstruction or a neurogenic bladder.

In children, RN is diagnosed mostly after UTI (acquired RN) or during follow-up for antenatally diagnosed hydronephrosis with no prior UTI (congenital RN). The acquired RN is more common in female children, whereas the congenital RN is more common in male children. This observation in children might help explain the differences in the clinical presentation of RN in adults, with males presenting mostly with hypertension, proteinuria and progressive renal failure (as compared with females, who present mostly with recurrent UTI and who generally have a better outcome). Known risk factors for RN include the severity of VUR, recurrent UTI, and bladder-bowel dysfunction; younger age and delay in treatment of UTI are believed to be other risk factors. Management of VUR is controversial and includes antimicrobial prophylaxis, surgical intervention or surveillance only. No evidence-based guidelines exist for appropriate follow-up of patients with RN.

VUR is graded I–IV as follows:

I   Reflux into the distal ureters
II   Reflux into the upper collecting system with no dilatation of the upper tract
III As for Grade II but with minor blunting of the calyces
IV   Reflux with hydroureter and calyceal dilatation
V   Reflux with massive dilatation of the ureter and upper tract.

VUR graded from I to III often resolves spontaneously as the child grows, but early recognition is important, as low-dose antibiotic cover is usually recommended to reduce the risk of permanent parenchymal damage. Surgical correction is usually reserved for children with severe reflux – this is commonly done by re-implantation of the ureters.

Reference

Mattoo TK. Vesicoureteral reflux and reflux nephropathy. *Adv Chronic Kidney Dis*. 2011; **18**(5): 348–54.

Case B

History

A 32-year-old woman investigated for early satiety; ultrasound showed focal lesion in the liver

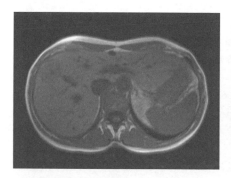

Figure i In-phase MRI

Figure ii Pre-contrast VIBE MRI

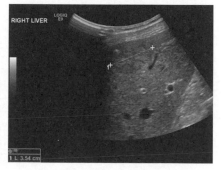

Figure iii Arterial phase VIBE MRI

Figure iv Ultrasound of the liver, right lobe

Observations and interpretation

Liver MRI with hepatocyte-specific contrast agent (axial T2 HASTE, in and out of phase, VIBE pre contrast, arterial phase and 10 minutes post contrast):

- well-defined mass in segment 8/5;
- the lesion is difficult to delineate on the unenhanced images;
- the lesion shows intense arterial enhancement with a non-enhancing central scar;
- enhancement does not wash out and the lesion shows enhancement during the liver specific phase of the examination;
- the lesion has benign characteristics;

- the rest of the liver is unremarkable bar simple hepatic cysts;
- no lymphadenopathy or other abnormality seen.

US:
- 3 cm lesion in the right lobe of the liver is almost isoechoic to normal parenchyma;
- lesion causes minor mass effect and is slightly heterogenous.

Main diagnosis
Typical focal nodular hyperplasia (FNH) – these are very typical imaging appearances for the benign pathology FNH

Differential diagnoses
- Adenoma, atypical haemangioma, hepatocellular carcinoma, atypical hypervascular metastases (these are all very unlikely, not only on the imaging criteria but also in the clinical context of a young female patient with a normal background liver)

Further management
- For discussion at the Hepatobiliary MDT meeting
- Need to enquire if the patient is taking the oral contraceptive pill or other hormone based medications
- For radiological follow-up as, although benign, these lesions are occasionally excised if they grow rapidly or become haemorrhagic
- This is probably an incidental finding, as is unlikely to be causing satiety issues; continue investigation of these symptoms

Discussion
FNH is a hamartomatous malformation and is the second most common benign liver tumour after hemangioma. It has no malignant potential. It is most commonly found in young adult women. FNH is classified into two types: classic (80% of cases) and non-classic (20%). Distinction between FNH and other hypervascular liver lesions such as adenoma, hepatocellular carcinoma and hypervascular metastases is obviously vital. An asymptomatic patient with FNH diagnosed on imaging does not usually require biopsy or surgery. Patients on oral contraceptives are usually advised to discontinue them, as use of oral contraceptives can cause the lesions to grow and is associated with a higher risk of haemorrhage. Haemorrhage is rare but a haemorrhagic rupture is a potentially life-threatening complication. Surgery is very rarely required – haemorrhage can be treated by

interventional radiology and only occasionally are large/growing or pedunculated masses excised.

Classic FNH is characterised by the presence of abnormal nodular architecture, malformed vessels and bile duct proliferation. Non-classic FNH lesions lack either nodular abnormal architecture or malformed vessels but they always show bile duct proliferation.

At imaging studies, typical and atypical lesions can often be distinguished on the basis of morphology, the appearance of the lesion relative to the surrounding liver on unenhanced images, the vascularity of the lesion, and the presence of any diffuse parenchymal liver disease. Ultrasound may often be the initial imaging modality that indicates a focal liver lesion. Typical FNH can be diagnosed with confidence at CT or MRI imaging.

At ultrasound, typical FNH is often not well visualised and can be very similar to the background parenchyma. There may be only a subtle change in echogenicity compared with the surrounding normal liver parenchyma. The conspicuity of the lesions at ultrasound may improve with a relatively large or prominent central scar. Some lesions may show a hypoechoic halo surrounding the lesion. This halo most likely represents compressed hepatic parenchyma or vessels surrounding the lesion. The halo may be more prominent in a liver with steatosis. The outer contours of the lesions may be well defined, although the internal structure of FNH, including the central scar, is often not well visualised. Use of color and power Doppler ultrasound may add information concerning the vascularity of the suspected FNH. In addition, use of ultrasound contrast media to characterise FNH has been shown to be useful.

Contrast-enhanced CT is a useful tool in the characterisation of focal liver lesions. However, because of radiation risk, particularly in younger patients, MRI may the cross-sectional modality of choice. Typically a triple-phase protocol is utilised comprising pre-contrast, arterial and portal venous phase imaging. At unenhanced CT, the lesions usually show a lobulated contour and are either hypoattenuating or isoattenuating to the surrounding liver. In the arterial phase, the lesions become hyperattenuating because of the homogeneous intense enhancement of the entire lesion, except the central scar. In the portal and later phases, the lesions become more isoattenuating and the surrounding liver and the central scar may show some enhancement.

MRI has higher sensitivity and specificity for FNH than ultrasonography or contrast-enhanced CT. Classic FNH is iso- or hypointense on T1-weighted images, is slightly hyper- or isointense on T2-weighted images, and has a hyperintense central scar on T2-weighted images. FNH demonstrates intense homogeneous enhancement during the arterial phase and can demonstrate delayed enhancement of the central scar. Familiarity with the proper MRI technique and the spectrum of MRI findings is essential for correct diagnosis of FNH.

Non-classic or atypical FNH is broadly divided into three subtypes: (1) telangiectatic FNH, (2) FNH with cytologic atypia and (3) mixed hyperplastic and adenomatous FNH. Telangiectatic FNH is most commonly associated with oral contraceptives and usually does not demonstrate a central scar. Atypical FNH may appear as a large lesion or is sometimes multiple in location. The lesion may show less intense enhancement, an atypical appearance or non-enhancement or absence of the central scar and pseudocapsular enhancement on delayed images. In these cases, it may be difficult to differentiate atypical FNH from benign and malignant lesions such as adenoma, hepatocellular carcinoma, fibrolamellar carcinoma and hypervascular hepatic metastases. This is where interval imaging or biopsy are useful.

Reference

Hussain SM, Terkivatan T, Zondervan PE, *et al.* Focal nodular hyperplasia: findings at state-of-the-art MR imaging, US, CT, and pathologic analysis. *Radiographics.* 2004; **24**(1): 3–17; discussion 18–19.

Case C

History

A 35-year-old with pain in the right breast

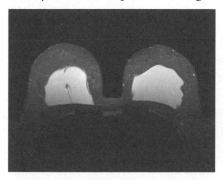

Figure i Axial STIR MRI

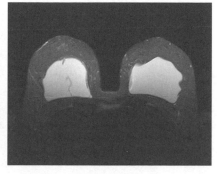

Figure ii Axial STIR MRI

Observations and interpretation

MRI of the breasts (STIR axial):

- bilateral submammary silicone implants are present;
- anteroposterior diameter of the right implant is greater than the left and it adopts a more spherical shape;
- 'noose sign' in the right breast superomedially;
- small amount of fluid surrounds the right implant;
- left implant appears normal;
- incidental radial folds in the right implant;
- no significant lesions outside the capsule identified.

Main diagnosis

Intracapsular rupture of the right implant without collapse, with no evidence of extracapsular rupture

Differential diagnoses

None

Further management

Referral to a breast surgeon/breast clinic

Discussion

Breast implants are becoming increasingly common. Most are implanted for augmentation purposes but a significant minority are patients who have undergone reconstructive procedures after breast surgery. Although many different types of implants are available, the majority are silicone based.

Assessment of breast lesions in patients with implants can be challenging. Not only is the breast tissue more difficult to image but also the patient may have complications from the implants themselves. The major complications of breast implants are post-procedural haematoma, infection, capsule contraction, rupture and silicone granulomas.

After an implant is inserted, the body forms a fibrous scar or capsule around the implant. This is a normal reaction to a foreign body but can cause contraction of the implant and can become symptomatic. Occasionally this capsule has to be manually broken down to relieve symptoms. Implant rupture is a very important complication to recognise, as this usually requires removal of the implant. Rupture can be intra- or extracapsular and can result in total, partial or no collapse of the shell. When the fibrous capsule is intact, implant ruptures are contained and referred to as intracapsular – this occurs in up to 90% of cases. Extracapsular ruptures result in extrusion of silicone into the adjacent breast tissue. This can cause inflammatory reactions and can potentially migrate to other parts of the body. Importantly, extracapsular silicone can cause confusion when investigating other focal lesions of the breast.

Imaging findings of a ruptured silicone implant vary according to the modality. On mammography, silicone density masses outside the implant is the only reliable sign of extracapsular rupture; intracapsular ruptures are obviously very difficult to delineate on mammography. With ultrasound the presence of low-level internal echoes and pairs/groups of linear internal echoes called 'doublets' or 'stepladders' can reliably indicate intracapsular rupture. Extracapsular rupture on ultrasound can create a 'snowstorm' effect. MRI is the most reliable way of assessing implant rupture; curvilinear decreased signal intensity within the implant known as the 'linguini sign' is often seen and droplets of fluid within the gel can also indicate rupture. The presence of low signal within the implant in the shape of an inverted 'teardrop' or 'noose' is a fairly specific sign for incomplete rupture. Of note radial folds emanating from the surface of the implant do not suggest rupture and are an incidental finding.

References

Berg WA, Caskey CI, Hamper UM, *et al.* Diagnosing breast implant rupture with MR imaging, US, and mammography. *Radiographics*. 1993; **13**(6): 1323–36.

Yang N, Muradali D. The augmented breast: a pictorial review of the abnormal and unusual. *AJR Am J Roentgenol*. 2011; **196**(4): W451–60.

Case D

History

A 64-year-old male with difficulty walking

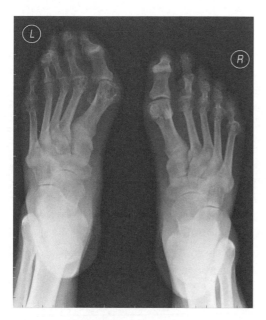

Figure i Radiograph of the feet

Observations and interpretation

Bilateral feet radiograph:

- number of abnormalities seen within the feet;
- periarticular cysts affecting the metatarsophalangeal joints, with subluxation of the left first, second and third metatarsophalangeal joints and narrowed joint spaces;
- no soft tissue swelling or calicification;
- the midfoot appears spared.

Main diagnosis

Appearances are of a bilateral symmetric erosive arthropathy, the most likely of which is rheumatoid arthritis.

Differential diagnoses

Other erosive arthropathies

Further management

Review of previous imaging for any progression and discussion with Rheumatology

Discussion

Rheumatoid arthritis is a chronic systemic condition of the synovium of multifactorial aetiology. Approximately 1% of the global population is affected, with females more than males. Early diagnosis is important to allow prompt treatment to modify the course of the disease and prevent the severely disabling late complications.

The disease is centred on the synovium, with tendon sheaths also affected. In the course of the synovial inflammation, the adjacent structures including bones, tendons, capsule and ligaments are also affected. The bone is affected initially at the 'bare area', between the insertion of the fibrous capsule and the cartilage, where the bone is only covered by synovium.

The key pathology involved is synovial hyperplasia, which forms into pannus. This is initiated by pro-inflammatory cytokines and immune cells. Subsequent hyperaemia and inactivity related to pain, leads to collateral bone damage. The synovium is infiltrated by inflammatory cells, followed by the articular cartilage and bone being degraded by enzymes, secreted by the pro-inflammatory cells. Loose bodies may form which contribute to the inflammation at the joints. The sequelae of untreated rheumatoid arthritis include; ankylosis, deformity and severe secondary osteoarthritis.

Early on, the bone changes are not apparent, as the disease is synovial-based. Therefore, ultrasound and MRI are preferable for detecting the presence of periarticular erosions, tenosynovitis (particularly of extensor carpi ulnaris), bursitis and inflammatory bone marrow oedema. Early signs on plain radiographs are; juxtaarticular osteopaenia and irregular cortical endplates, however, there are other non-specific features, including joint space widening, soft tissue swelling and fat pad elevation.

It is generally preferred to image any symptomatic joints, such as hands, wrists or feet, as any joint may be involved at any one time and there is potentially improved diagnostic yield from imaging a symptomatic joint. At the stage where synovitis only is present, the disease is potentially reversible by disease modifying anti-rheumatic drugs.

Months after the onset of the disease, subcortical cysts develop, which in association with an inflammatory process, are typically seen in an eccentric location, with irregular margins and in groups of more than three. Progression of the disease leads to destruction of articular cartilage and joint space narrowing.

It is important to remember that RA can be a systemic condition, and have extra-articular complications, such as anaemia, vasculitis, pericarditis, hepatosplenomegaly, rheumatic rash, fever and others.

References

Jacobson JA, Girish G, Jiang Y, *et al*. Radiographic evaluation of arthritis: inflammatory conditions. *Radiology*. 2008; **248**(2): 378–89.

Jacobson JA, Girish G, Jiang Y, *et al*. Radiographic evaluation of arthritis: degenerative joint disease and variations. *Radiology*. 2008; **248**(3): 737–47.

Case E
History
A 73-year-old with cognitive decline

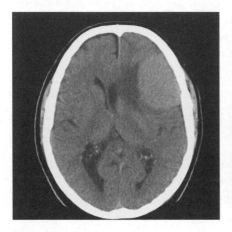

Figure i Pre-contrast CT   **Figure ii** Post-contrast CT

Observations and interpretation
Pre- and post-contrast CT of the head:
- on the non-contrast scan, there is a large hyperdense lesion within the left frontal region;
- there is a small amount of surrounding vasogenic oedema, with local mass effect causing effacement and displacement of the left frontal horn, effacement of sulci of the left cerebral hemisphere and midline shift;
- the basal cisterns are patent;
- there is also mild left transtentorial herniation, consistent with raised intracranial pressure;
- post contrast, the lesion demonstrates homogenous enhancement, with a broad-based dural attachment and a dural tail;
- no further lesions are seen;
- on bone windows, there is slight irregularity of the adjacent inner table in keeping with hyperostosis.

Main diagnosis
The appearances are of an extra-axial lesion causing significant local mass effect, most likely a meningioma.

Differential diagnoses
None

Further management
Urgent report to clinical team and referral to Neurosurgery for definitive management

Discussion
It can sometimes be difficult to distinguish between intra- and extra-axial lesions; however, it will help with forming a list of differential diagnoses. Extra-axial structures include those outside the brain (arachnoid, meninges, dural sinuses) and the ventricular system. Features seen with extra-axial masses include inward compression or 'buckling' of white matter with preservation of the grey-white matter interface. Intra-axial lesions have features including expansion of the white matter and blurring of the grey-white matter interface.

Meningiomas are the most common extra-axial neoplasm, accounting for 15% of all intracranial neoplasms, with a peak age in the sixth decade. Women are more commonly affected, with a hormonal response by the tumour to increase in size during pregnancy. These lesions are generally slow growing and derive their vascular supply from the external carotid artery branches. The locations where meningiomas occur, in order of frequency, include parasagittal/convexity, splenoid wing, planum sphenoidale, parasellar cistern, intraventricular, tentorium and optic nerve sheath. Intraspinal lesions can also occur, most often in the thoracic spine.

There are typical appearances for meningiomas. On plain films (although skull radiographs are rarely performed), findings include focal sclerosis, prominent dural grooves from enlarged middle meningeal arteries and calcification. CT findings include a hyperdense mass, with variable surrounding oedema, intense homogenous enhancement post contrast, and hyperostosis of the inner table in approximately half of the cases. Calcification is seen in approximately a fifth of cases. MRI characteristics include isointense to hypointense to grey matter on T1 and isointense to hyperintense on T2. Heterogeneity may be seen due to the presence of vessels, cysts or calcification. Prominent pial vessel flow voids may be seen, confirming the extra-axial location. A broad dural base is also often seen, with adjacent dural thickening, the 'dural tail' seen in 60% of cases. A neurosurgical consideration is to assess for involvement of the dural sinuses, demonstrated as a reduction in the calibre of a dural sinus adjacent to a meningioma. Evaluation with MRI angiography or contrast angiography may be required.

Other extra-axial entities include haemangiopericytoma (previously known as angioblastic meningioma, which has a more aggressive pattern, including bone destruction, narrow dural attachement and propensity to metastasise), secondary central nervous system lymphoma (typically involving the leptomeninges), dural metastases (causing brain compression or venous sinus thrombosis, often secondary to breast, lung, prostate or renal malignancy with associated adjacent skull involvement).

Reference

Koeller KK. Central nervous system neoplasms and tumourlike masses. In: Brant WE, Helms CA. *Fundamentals of Diagnostic Radiology*. 3rd ed. Philadelphia, USA: Lippincott, Williams & Wilkins; 2007. pp. 122–55.

Case F

History

A 50-year-old male with epigastric pain

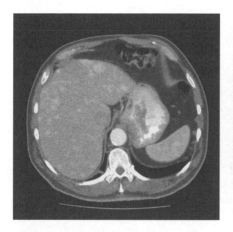

Figure i Arterial phase CT

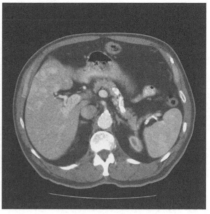

Figure ii Arterial phase CT

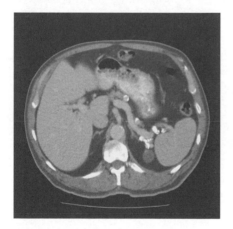

Figure iii Portal venous phase CT

Observations and interpretation

Arterial and portal venous phase CT of the chest, abdomen and pelvis:

- no mediastinal or hilar lymphadenopathy;
- heavily calcified left anterior descending artery;
- on arterial phase, there are multiple high-density areas within the liver, which become isodense to the liver during portal venous phase;
- the liver has a smooth capsule with no evidence of nodules;

- multiple calcified serpiginous calcified areas around the pancreas and spleen;
- uncomplicated infrarenal abdominal aortic aneurysm with mural haematoma;
- atrophic left kidney;
- normal right kidney, spleen, pancreas and bowel.

Main diagnosis

Intrahepatic arteriovenous malformations (AVMs) (background of hereditary haemorrhagic telangiectasia)

Differential diagnoses

- Hypervascular metastases secondary to neuroendocrine primary
- Multiple haemangiomas

Further management

- Review of previous imaging for any interval change
- Refer to interventional radiology in case embolisation is required

Discussion

As with anywhere in the body, vascular malformations can be subdivided into fast-flow (AVMs, arterioportal fistulas), slow-flow (portosystemic shunts, venous and lymphatic malformations) and combined forms. AVMs are defined as congenital abnormalities in the formation of blood vessels that shunt blood through direct arteriovenous connections. There is no abnormal neoplastic tissue found between the anomalous vessels, which is another cause of neovascularity.

The imaging appearance of hepatic AVMs overlaps with those of haemangiomas. On ultrasound, one would expect to find a collection of tortuous enlarged vessels, commonly located in one lobe of the liver, with high peak Doppler shifts in both arteries and veins, low arterial resistive index and increased pulsatility of veins. Unenhanced CT may reveal hypoattenuating lesions, which enhance avidly in the arterial or early portal venous phase, with rapid washout of contrast in the later phases. MRI can assist in distinguishing between an AVM and a haemangioma. Absent delayed uptake of contrast around the hypertrophic vessels make AVM more likely. Angiography demonstrates poor regional definition of the lesion, with arteriovenous shunting, puddling of contrast material in the vascular spaces and no parenchymal blush.

Hereditary haemorrhagic telangiectasia is a rare autosomal dominant, multisystem vascular disorder that occurs in approximately 1 in 10 000 of the population. The key feature is of angiodysplastic lesions, with direct communication between arteries and veins of different sizes with no capillary network in between. The sequelae include bleeding and shunting. Typically, the skin, lungs and mucous membranes are involved, but any organ may be affected. Hepatic involvement occurs in approximately 75% of affected individuals, and quantification of hepatic disease burden can be useful for prognosis and treatment.

There are a variety of abdominal findings that may be seen in patients with hereditary haemorrhagic telangiectasia. In the liver, the most commonly seen lesions are telangiectases (hypervascular, rounded masses, in the shape of an asterisk, usually a few millimeters in diameter; telangiectases are hyperattenuating in the arterial phase and isodense in the portal venous phase). If these telangiectases coalesce, the resulting lesion is known as a large confluent vascular mass, which may demonstrate contrast enhancement into the venous phase. Hepatic perfusion abnormalities can occur, which are best seen in the arterial and early venous phases. Hepatic shunts can also occur, with arteriovenous (hepatic artery to hepatic vein) being the most common. Elsewhere in the abdomen, other vascular anomalies can be seen in other organs, including pancreatic AVMs, splenic artery aneurysms.

References

Gallego C, Miralles M, Marin C, *et al.* Congenital hepatic shunts. *Radiographics.* 2004; **24**(3): 755–72.

Siddiki H, Doherty MG, Fletcher JG, *et al.* Abdominal findings in hereditary hemorrhagic telangiectasia: pictorial essay on 2D and 3D findings with isotropic multiphase CT. *Radiographics.* 2008; **28**(1): 171–84.

Index